From Diagnosis to

DAILY LIVING

A Compassionate Guide

to Alzheimer's

CONTENTS

Introduction 3

Definition and overview of Alzheimer's disease 5

Importance of Understanding Alzheimer's Disease 19

Understanding Alzheimer's Disease 29

Historical Perspective and Discovery 31

Causes and Risk Factors 40

Common Symptoms and Manifestations 52

Diagnostic procedures and tests for Alzheimer's Disease 69

Current treatment options and medications 76

Non-pharmacological interventions and therapies 80

Impact on Patients and Caregivers 87

Introduction

Consider a society in which familiar faces blur, cherished memories fade like photographs left in the sun, and even the simplest chores become difficult obstacles. This is the reality for millions of people suffering with Alzheimer's disease, a degenerative neurological disorder that robs us of our fundamental identity. It's a silent thief who steals people's independence and leaves loved ones to deal with a future they never envisaged.

For many, the first signs of Alzheimer's might be a misplaced car key, a forgotten appointment, or the struggle to recall a familiar name. These seemingly minor incidents can be the first ripples on a pond, a harbinger of a storm that will reshape lives forever. Yet, beneath the surface of this disease lies a complex story, a biological puzzle waiting to be unraveled.

This book is your guide on that journey. We'll delve into the science behind Alzheimer's, exploring the intricate workings of the brain and the cellular changes that lead to this devastating illness. We'll unpack the symptoms, from the initial forgetfulness to the later stages of confusion and disorientation. Understanding these signs is crucial for early detection, which can empower individuals and families to make informed decisions about care.

But Alzheimer's is more than just a medical condition; it's a human story. We'll meet individuals living with the disease, hearing their experiences in their own words. We'll explore the challenges faced by caregivers, the unsung heroes who provide unwavering support and navigate the labyrinth of emotions that come with watching a loved one disappear piece by piece.

This journey won't be without hope. We'll explore the world of cutting-edge research, where scientists are tirelessly searching for a cure and better treatment options. We'll highlight the ongoing clinical trials that offer a glimmer of light for the future. We'll discuss lifestyle choices that may help reduce the risk of developing the disease, empowering you to take control of your own brain health.

This book is not just for those directly affected by Alzheimer's. It's for everyone who knows someone who forgets, who struggles to find the right words, or who simply fears the prospect of losing their memories. It's for those who want to understand, to empathize, and to make a difference in the fight against this relentless disease.

As you turn the pages, you'll gain the knowledge and tools needed to navigate the complexities of Alzheimer's. You'll learn how to support those living with the disease, how to advocate for better care, and how to stay informed about the latest advancements. Together, we can build a future where Alzheimer's no longer steals memories, but where hope and resilience prevail.

This is more than just a book; it's a call to action. Let's embark on this journey together, one step, one memory, at a time.

Definition and overview of Alzheimer's disease

- **What is Alzheimer's Disease?**

Have you ever walked into a room and forgotten why you were there? Misplaced your keys for a moment, only to find them in the usual spot? These occasional memory lapses are a normal part of aging. But what if these forgetful moments become more frequent and severe? What if they begin to disrupt your daily life and cast a shadow over your independence? This could be a sign of Alzheimer's disease, a progressive neurological disorder that robs individuals of their memories and cognitive abilities.

The line between normal forgetfulness and the beginnings of Alzheimer's can sometimes feel blurry. We all experience occasional memory lapses as we age. Forgetting a name here or there, struggling to recall a specific detail from a conversation – these are usually nothing to worry about.

However, Alzheimer's disease goes beyond occasional forgetfulness. It's a progressive disease, meaning it worsens over time. The hallmark symptoms of Alzheimer's are:

Memory loss that disrupts daily life: This is not just forgetting a name or appointment. It's forgetting how to perform familiar tasks like cooking, driving, or managing finances.

Difficulty with reasoning and problem-solving: Simple tasks like balancing a checkbook or following a recipe become increasingly challenging.

Challenges with language: Struggling to find the right words, difficulty following conversations, or repeating oneself frequently are all signs of language difficulties associated with Alzheimer's.

Changes in personality and behavior: Individuals with Alzheimer's may become withdrawn, anxious, or even aggressive. They may experience sleep disturbances or wanderlust.

- **The Underlying Pathology: Plaques and Tangles**

While the exact causes of Alzheimer's are still under investigation, scientists have identified some key players in the disease process. The brains of individuals with Alzheimer's show a buildup of abnormal proteins:

Amyloid plaques: These are sticky clusters of protein fragments that form between nerve cells in the brain.

Neurofibrillary tangles: These are twisted strands of another protein that accumulate inside nerve cells.

These plaques and tangles disrupt communication between brain cells and eventually lead to the death of those cells. The areas of the brain most affected by these changes are the ones responsible for memory, thinking, language, and reasoning. This explains why these very functions decline as Alzheimer's progresses.

Alzheimer's disease doesn't manifest the same way in everyone. The rate of progression can vary greatly, with some individuals experiencing a more rapid decline than others. There are also different stages of Alzheimer's, each with its own set of symptoms:

Early Stage: This stage is often characterized by mild memory loss, difficulty concentrating, and challenges with planning and organization.

Middle Stage: As the disease progresses, memory loss becomes more severe. Individuals may struggle with daily tasks like dressing or bathing. Confusion and personality changes become more noticeable.

Late Stage: In the late stages of Alzheimer's, individuals lose the ability to speak, care for themselves, and eventually, respond to their environment.

- **It's not just about memory**

While memory loss is often the most recognizable symptom of Alzheimer's, it's important to remember that the disease affects more than just our ability to recall past experiences. People with Alzheimer's may also experience:

Vision problems: Depth perception and spatial awareness can be impaired.

Loss of balance and coordination: This can increase the risk of falls and injuries.

Mood swings and depression: The frustration and confusion associated with Alzheimer's can lead to emotional distress.

Changes in sleep patterns: Individuals with Alzheimer's may experience sleep disturbances, including insomnia or excessive daytime sleepiness.

Alzheimer's disease presents a unique set of challenges for both the individual diagnosed and their loved ones. The progressive nature of the disease means facing a future filled with uncertainty. The fear of losing oneself, the burden on caregivers, and the emotional toll on families are all realities that those living with Alzheimer's must confront. Unfortunately, this disease is becoming increasingly common. As the population ages, the number of people diagnosed with Alzheimer's is expected to rise significantly. Understanding the disease, its symptoms, and the impact it has on individuals and families is crucial.

While there is currently no cure for Alzheimer's, there are treatment options available that can help manage symptoms and improve quality of life. Research is ongoing, and scientists are actively searching for ways to prevent, slow the progression of, and ultimately cure this devastating disease.

- **The Impact of Alzheimer's: A Ripple Effect**

Alzheimer's disease casts a long shadow, impacting not just the individual diagnosed but also their loved ones and society as a whole. Understanding the prevalence of this disease is the first step in recognizing its far-reaching consequences.

Alzheimer's disease is the most common form of dementia, a general term for memory loss and cognitive decline that interferes with daily life. According to the Alzheimer's Association, nearly 7 million Americans are currently living with Alzheimer's. This number is projected to rise to nearly 13 million by 2050, highlighting the alarming growth of this disease.

For the individual diagnosed with Alzheimer's, the disease represents a progressive erosion of self. The initial forgetfulness can evolve into a complete loss of independence as daily tasks become increasingly challenging. Simple things like managing finances, preparing meals, or taking medications become insurmountable hurdles. The ability to communicate effectively can deteriorate, leading to frustration and isolation.

The burden of caring for someone with Alzheimer's often falls on family members. Witnessing a loved one lose their memories, personality, and independence can be incredibly heartbreaking. Spouses, children, and siblings become caregivers, juggling complex medical needs alongside their own emotional well-being. The stress of caregiving can lead to depression, anxiety, and social isolation for families.

Alzheimer's disease represents a significant financial burden on families and society as a whole. The cost of care, including medical expenses, assisted living facilities, and home care, can be astronomical. This financial strain can deplete life savings and leave families struggling to make ends meet. On a national level, Alzheimer's disease and other forms of dementia are projected to cost the United States nearly $1 trillion in 2050.

The ripple effect of Alzheimer's extends beyond families and healthcare systems. The loss of a loved one's cognitive abilities can have a profound impact on social interactions. Individuals with Alzheimer's may withdraw from social activities, leading to feelings of loneliness and isolation. Additionally, the disease can strain relationships with friends and extended family members who may struggle to understand or interact with someone in the later stages of the disease.

The growing prevalence of Alzheimer's demands a collective response. Raising awareness about the disease is crucial for several reasons:

Early Detection: Early diagnosis allows individuals with Alzheimer's to access treatment options and plan for the future. By recognizing the early signs and symptoms, families can make informed decisions about care.

Increased Funding for Research: Greater public awareness about the impact of Alzheimer's can lead to increased research funding. This is essential for developing new treatments, finding a cure, and ultimately, combating this devastating illness.

Building a Support System: Raising awareness can help create a more supportive environment for individuals and families living with Alzheimer's. This may involve establishing support groups, providing educational resources, and advocating for policies that support caregivers.

A Shared Challenge: Looking Towards the future the impact of Alzheimer's is undeniable. However, by understanding the challenges it poses, we can begin to develop solutions.

- **The Stages of Alzheimer's**

Alzheimer's disease is a progressive illness, meaning its symptoms worsen over time. The progression can vary significantly from person to person, but there are generally three recognized stages: early, middle, and late. Understanding these stages can help individuals, families, and caregivers anticipate the challenges ahead and plan for the future.

- **Early Stage (Mild Cognitive Impairment)**

The early stage of Alzheimer's can be a subtle and confusing time. Symptoms are often mild and may be mistaken for normal signs of aging. Here's what you might observe:

Increased forgetfulness: This is often the most noticeable symptom. Individuals may forget names, appointments, or conversations.

Difficulty with multitasking: Following complex instructions or juggling multiple tasks at once can become challenging.

Mild problems with planning and organization: Planning meals, paying bills, or managing finances may require more effort.

Misplacing belongings: Keys, wallets, or glasses may be misplaced more frequently.

It's important to note that not everyone with mild memory problems has Alzheimer's. Other health conditions or medications can also cause similar symptoms. However, if these difficulties become persistent and interfere with daily life, a doctor's evaluation is crucial to rule out other causes and determine if Alzheimer's might be present.

- **Middle Stage (Moderate Cognitive Decline)**

As the disease progresses, the symptoms become more pronounced. In the middle stage, individuals with Alzheimer's may experience:

More significant memory loss: Forgetting recent events, familiar faces, or even personal information becomes more common.

Difficulty with communication: Finding the right words or following conversations can be challenging. Individuals may repeat themselves frequently.

Disorientation and confusion: Getting lost in familiar places, struggling to tell time, or having difficulty understanding the date can occur.

Changes in personality and behavior: Individuals may become withdrawn, anxious, or even aggressive. Sleep disturbances and wandering are also common in this stage.

Daily living activities become increasingly difficult at this stage. Individuals may need assistance with bathing, dressing, and preparing meals. The burden of care often falls on family members who must learn to manage the patient's needs while coping with their own emotional challenges.

- **Late Stage (Severe Cognitive Decline)**

The late stage of Alzheimer's is marked by a significant decline in cognitive and physical abilities. Individuals may experience:

Severe memory loss: They may forget who they are, where they are, and even how to perform basic tasks.

Loss of communication skills: Verbal communication may become limited to simple words or phrases. Nonverbal methods of communication become more important.

Complete dependence on caregivers: Individuals require assistance with all aspects of daily living, including eating, dressing, and toileting.

Increased physical limitations: Muscle weakness, difficulty walking, and swallowing problems may occur.

In the late stage, comfort care becomes the primary focus. The goal is to manage pain, maintain comfort, and ensure the emotional well-being of the individual.

- **It's a Spectrum, Not a Straight Line**

It's important to remember that these stages are a general framework. The progression of Alzheimer's can vary significantly from person to person. Some individuals may move quickly through the stages, while others may remain stable in a particular stage for a longer period. Additionally, the specific symptoms experienced can vary. Some people may struggle more with memory loss, while others may have more prominent personality changes.

Understanding the stages of Alzheimer's can be helpful, but it's crucial to remember that every individual with this disease is unique. The most effective care plan should be tailored to the specific needs and abilities of the person diagnosed. Working with a healthcare team, including doctors, nurses, and social workers, can ensure that individuals with Alzheimer's receive the support and resources they need at each stage of their journey.

- **The Hallmarks of Alzheimer's: Plaques and Tangles – A Cellular Mystery**

Imagine the intricate network of the brain as a bustling highway system. Billions of nerve cells, called neurons, act as the highways, communicating with each other to carry out all the functions that make us who we are – from remembering our loved ones to solving complex problems. In Alzheimer's disease, this finely tuned system gets disrupted by the presence of abnormal proteins that accumulate in the brain, like roadblocks hindering smooth traffic flow. These roadblocks are known as plaques and tangles, and they are considered the hallmarks of Alzheimer's disease.

- **Plaques: Sticky Deposits Disrupting Communication**

One of the key players in Alzheimer's is a protein called beta-amyloid. Normally, this protein is broken down and eliminated from the brain. However, in Alzheimer's disease, fragments of beta-amyloid clump together, forming sticky plaques that accumulate between nerve cells. Think of these plaques like debris littering the highway, obstructing the pathways between neurons.

The presence of plaques disrupts communication in the brain. Neurons rely on chemical messengers called neurotransmitters to communicate with each other. Plaques can interfere with the release and reception of these neurotransmitters, hindering the brain's ability to transmit information.

- **Tangles: Twisted Proteins Inside Cells**

Another culprit in Alzheimer's disease is a protein called tau. In a healthy brain, tau acts like a scaffold, providing structural support for neurons. However, in Alzheimer's, tau protein undergoes a change, becoming twisted and tangled. These tangled tau proteins accumulate inside nerve cells, disrupting their internal structure and function.

Imagine these tangles as frayed wires within the neurons. Just like faulty wiring disrupts the functioning of an appliance, tangled tau proteins prevent neurons from working properly. This can lead to the death of nerve cells, further contributing to the decline in cognitive function observed in Alzheimer's disease.

Scientists are still trying to understand the exact relationship between plaques and tangles in Alzheimer's disease. It's unclear whether the buildup of plaques triggers the formation of tangles, or vice versa. It's also possible that both processes occur independently, but ultimately contribute to the decline in brain function.

- **More Than Just Plaques and Tangles**

While plaques and tangles are considered the hallmarks of Alzheimer's disease, it's important to note that other factors are likely involved. Inflammation, oxidative stress (damage caused by free radicals), and impaired blood flow to the brain may also play a role in the disease process.

Understanding the role of plaques and tangles is crucial for developing new treatments for Alzheimer's disease. Researchers are exploring various approaches:

Targeting Beta-amyloid: Some medications aim to prevent the formation of plaques or to clear existing plaques from the brain.

Targeting Tau: Other therapies focus on preventing tau protein from tangling or promoting its breakdown.

Combination Therapies: Researchers are also exploring the possibility of combining different approaches to target both plaques and tangles.

While plaques and tangles are the focus of much research, it's important to remember that Alzheimer's disease affects the whole person. The next sections of this book will delve deeper into the symptoms of the disease, the impact it has on individuals and families, and the ongoing search for a cure. We'll also explore ways to support those living with Alzheimer's disease and advocate for better care and resources.

- **The Mystery of Alzheimer's: Unveiling the Unknown**

Alzheimer's disease is a thief of memories, a relentless force that steals the very essence of who we are. While the presence of plaques and tangles in the brain is a defining feature of the disease, the exact causes of this devastating illness remain shrouded in mystery. Scientists around the world are working tirelessly to unravel this puzzle, but many questions linger, beckoning us to delve deeper.

Age is the biggest risk factor for Alzheimer's disease, but genetics also plays a role. Having a close relative with Alzheimer's increases your risk of developing the disease. Scientists have identified specific genes that are linked to an increased risk, but these genes don't guarantee that someone will develop the disease. It's more like a loaded gun – the genes may increase the risk, but other factors are likely needed to pull the trigger.

While genetics play a part, Alzheimer's is not simply a predetermined fate. Environmental factors also influence your risk of developing the disease. Head injuries, chronic health conditions like diabetes and high blood pressure, and certain lifestyle choices may contribute. This suggests that there may be ways to modify our environment and behaviors to potentially reduce our risk.

Research suggests that a healthy lifestyle may play a role in protecting against Alzheimer's. Maintaining a balanced diet, regular exercise, and engaging in mentally stimulating activities like learning a new language or playing chess may help keep your brain sharp. Additionally, managing stress and getting enough sleep are crucial for overall brain health.

Chronic inflammation in the body has been linked to various health conditions, including Alzheimer's disease. Scientists are investigating the possibility that chronic inflammation may contribute to the formation of plaques and tangles. Understanding this connection could lead to new interventions aimed at reducing inflammation and potentially slowing the progression of the disease

Recent research has shed light on the fascinating link between the gut microbiome and brain health. The trillions of bacteria living in our gut may play a role in cognitive function and influence the risk of neurodegenerative diseases like Alzheimer's. This opens up a new avenue of exploration, with scientists asking whether manipulating the gut microbiome could have a positive impact on brain health.

As we delve deeper into the world of Alzheimer's, the more we realize how much we still don't know. Some unanswered questions continue to intrigue scientists:

- **What triggers the buildup of plaques and tangles? Is it a single event or a combination of factors?**

- **Is there a specific order in which plaques and tangles develop? Does one trigger the formation of the other?**

- **Are there other factors besides plaques and tangles that contribute to the disease?**

- **Why does Alzheimer's affect some people more severely than others? Is it related to individual genetic variations or environmental exposures?**

Importance of Understanding Alzheimer's Disease

Empowering Individuals: Taking Control in the Face of Alzheimer's

A diagnosis of Alzheimer's disease can feel like a heavy blow, but knowledge is power. Understanding the disease empowers individuals to take control of their situation, navigate the complexities of their journey, and make informed decisions about their care. Here's how understanding Alzheimer's can benefit individuals:

Early Detection and Diagnosis: A Window of Opportunity

Early detection of Alzheimer's disease allows individuals to access treatment options and plan for the future. Many countries are implementing initiatives to promote early detection:

The United Kingdom's Dementia Friends program educates the public about the signs of dementia and encourages open conversations about the disease. This initiative has empowered individuals to seek help sooner, leading to earlier diagnoses. The United States National Alzheimer's Plan includes a focus on early detection and diagnosis. This plan calls for increased access to cognitive assessments and the development of new screening tools.

By recognizing the early signs of forgetfulness, difficulty concentrating, or changes in behavior, individuals can talk to their doctor about a cognitive assessment. Early diagnosis allows individuals to:

Start treatment options: While there is no cure for Alzheimer's, medications can help manage symptoms and improve quality of life.

Plan for the future: Individuals can make informed decisions about finances, legal matters, and long-term care options while they are still cognitively able to do so.

Participate in clinical trials: Early diagnosis opens doors for participation in clinical trials, which are crucial for developing new treatments and finding a cure.

Making Informed Decisions About Care: Your Voice Matters

Understanding Alzheimer's empowers individuals to be active participants in their own care. Here's how:

Understanding Treatment Options: Knowledge of available medications and their potential side effects allows individuals to work with their doctor to create a personalized treatment plan.

Researching Care Facilities: As the disease progresses, the need for assisted living or nursing home care may arise. Understanding the different care options and their associated costs empowers individuals to make informed choices.

Advocating for Preferences: Individuals with Alzheimer's can still express their preferences for care, even in the later stages. Understanding the disease helps them communicate these preferences to loved ones and caregivers.

Examples of Programs Promoting Informed Decision Making:

The Alzheimer's Association's https://www.alz.org/ website provides a wealth of information on caregiving, treatment options, and available resources.

The Netherlands' Mentorship Program for People with Dementia pairs individuals with trained mentors who can provide support and guidance throughout their journey with Alzheimer's.

Managing Symptoms and Maintaining Quality of Life

Living with Alzheimer's doesn't mean losing your quality of life. Understanding the disease allows individuals to develop strategies for managing symptoms and staying engaged in activities they enjoy.

Cognitive Strategies: Learning memory aids and organization techniques can help individuals cope with forgetfulness and maintain some degree of independence.

Physical Activity: Regular exercise has been shown to improve cognitive function and overall well-being for individuals with Alzheimer's.

Social Engagement: Staying connected with loved ones and participating in social activities, even in adapted ways, can help reduce isolation and improve mood.

Examples of Programs Supporting Quality of Life:

The Teepa Snow's Positive Approach to Care program emphasizes building relationships and respecting the personhood of individuals with dementia. This approach can help individuals feel valued and empowered.

The Music & Memory program utilizes personalized playlists to improve mood, memory, and communication for people with Alzheimer's.

By understanding Alzheimer's disease, individuals can become active participants in their own care journey. Early detection allows for a timely treatment plan, while knowledge empowers informed decision-making about care options. Finally, understanding symptoms empowers individuals to develop strategies for managing their condition and maintaining a fulfilling life.

Supporting Caregivers: The Unsung Heroes on the Frontlines of Alzheimer's

The burden of caring for someone with Alzheimer's disease often falls on loved ones – spouses, children, or siblings. These dedicated caregivers provide invaluable support, but the journey can be emotionally draining and physically demanding. Understanding Alzheimer's disease is crucial not just for individuals diagnosed but also for those who support them. Here's how knowledge empowers caregivers:

Understanding the Stages of the Disease: Knowing what to expect at each stage of Alzheimer's helps caregivers anticipate challenges and adapt their care approach accordingly.

Learning Effective Communication Strategies: As the disease progresses, communication can become difficult. Understanding the specific challenges faced by individuals with Alzheimer's allows caregivers to develop effective communication techniques.

Identifying Available Resources: Numerous organizations offer support groups, educational programs, and respite care options for caregivers. Knowing where to find these resources is essential for managing the demands of caregiving.

Examples of Programs Providing Practical Guidance: The Alzheimer's Association: https://www.alz.org/ offers a wealth of information on caregiving, including online resources, educational workshops, and support groups.

The Family Caregiver Alliance: https://www.caregiver.org/ provides a national network of support groups and educational programs for caregivers.

Building Resilience and Managing Stress:

Caregiving for someone with Alzheimer's can be a stressful and emotionally draining experience. Here's how understanding the disease can help caregivers build resilience and manage stress:

Managing Expectations: Understanding the progressive nature of the disease allows caregivers to set realistic expectations about their loved one's abilities.

Practicing Self-Care: Caregivers often neglect their own needs. Understanding the importance of self-care empowers them to prioritize their physical and mental well-being. This can include getting enough sleep, exercising regularly, and engaging in activities they enjoy.

Developing Coping Mechanisms: Learning relaxation techniques such as deep breathing or meditation can help caregivers manage stress and emotional strain.

Examples of Programs Supporting Caregiver Resilience: The Rosalynn Carter Institute for Caregivers: https://rosalynncarter.org/ provides training programs and resources to help caregivers develop coping mechanisms and build resilience.

The National Alliance for Caregiving: https://www.caregiving.org/ offers a variety of resources to help caregivers manage stress, such as online support groups and educational webinars.

Navigating the Emotional Journey:

Alzheimer's brings a wave of complex emotions for caregivers. Understanding the disease allows them to navigate this emotional rollercoaster and build a sense of acceptance.

Recognizing Normal Emotions: Caregivers may experience a range of emotions, including frustration, anger, guilt, and sadness. Understanding that these feelings are normal can be validating and alleviate self-blame.

Coping with Grief: As the disease progresses, caregivers may experience a sense of grief over the loss of their loved one's personality and independence. Knowledge of the grieving process can guide them through this difficult time.

Finding Support: Connecting with other caregivers who understand the challenges can provide invaluable emotional support and a sense of community.

Examples of Programs Supporting the Emotional Journey:

The Alzheimer's Association Dementia Support Groups: https://www.alz.org/help-support/community/support-groups provide a safe space for caregivers to share their experiences, receive emotional support, and connect with others on a similar journey.

The National Council on Aging's (NCOA) Caregiver Resource Center: https://www.ncoa.org/caregivers offers online resources and telephone support for caregivers experiencing emotional distress.

Fueling Research and Innovation: The Hope for a Brighter Future

Alzheimer's disease is a formidable opponent, but we are not without weapons in this fight. Research and innovation hold the key to unlocking new treatment options, exploring preventative strategies, and ultimately, finding a cure. Understanding the disease is crucial for fueling these efforts.

Identifying New Treatment Options:

The current medications for Alzheimer's primarily manage symptoms rather than stopping the progression of the disease. Understanding the underlying causes of Alzheimer's, such as the buildup of plaques and tangles in the brain, allows researchers to develop new treatment approaches:

Targeting Plaques and Tangles: Several promising therapies are being investigated that aim to prevent the formation of plaques or to clear existing plaques from the brain. Other research focuses on developing drugs that inhibit the formation of tangles or promote their breakdown.

Immunotherapy: This approach harnesses the body's immune system to attack the plaques and tangles in the brain. While still in early stages of development, immunotherapy holds promise for future treatment options.

Treating Underlying Conditions: Research suggests that addressing underlying health conditions like diabetes and high blood pressure may also be beneficial in managing Alzheimer's disease.

Examples of Research Initiatives:

The Alzheimer's Association International Conference (AAIC): [invalid URL removed] is a major platform for researchers to share their latest findings and advancements in Alzheimer's research.

The National Institute on Aging (NIA): [invalid URL removed] is a leading government agency funding research on Alzheimer's disease and other neurodegenerative conditions.

Exploring Preventative Strategies:

While there is no guaranteed way to prevent Alzheimer's, research suggests that adopting a healthy lifestyle may play a role in reducing your risk. Understanding the disease allows individuals to focus on:

Maintaining a Brain-Healthy Diet: Eating a balanced diet rich in fruits, vegetables, and whole grains may help protect brain health.

Regular Exercise: Physical activity has been shown to improve cognitive function and reduce the risk of developing dementia.

Cognitive Stimulation: Mentally stimulating activities like learning a new language, playing chess, or doing puzzles may help keep your brain sharp.

Managing Stress: Chronic stress can have a negative impact on brain health. Learning relaxation techniques such as yoga or meditation can help manage stress levels.

Examples of Preventative Programs:

The Alzheimer's Prevention Program (APP): [invalid URL removed] offers a research-based program that teaches participants lifestyle strategies to potentially reduce their risk of developing Alzheimer's disease.

The Finger Institutes for Health: [invalid URL removed] promotes brain health through educational programs and research initiatives focused on lifestyle interventions.

Working Towards a Cure:

The ultimate goal of Alzheimer's research is to find a cure that can halt or reverse the progression of the disease. Understanding the complex biological processes involved allows scientists to develop more targeted therapies:

Genetics and Personalized Medicine: Researching the link between genetics and Alzheimer's may pave the way for personalized medicine approaches, tailoring treatments based on an individual's specific genetic makeup.

Early Intervention: Detecting and diagnosing Alzheimer's at the earliest stages may allow for more effective treatment interventions before the disease progresses significantly.

Combination Therapies: Researchers are exploring the possibility of combining different treatment approaches to target various aspects of the disease process.

Examples of Research Funding Initiatives:

The Alzheimer's Association Advocacy Efforts: [invalid URL removed] work to secure increased government funding for Alzheimer's research.

Philanthropic Organizations: Many foundations and organizations dedicated to Alzheimer's research raise funds to support ongoing research initiatives.

The Power of Knowledge: Fueling Hope

Understanding Alzheimer's disease empowers not just individuals and caregivers but also the entire research community. By unraveling the mysteries of this disease, we can fuel innovation, identify new treatment options, explore preventative strategies, and ultimately, work towards a cure. This collective effort offers a glimmer of hope for a future free from Alzheimer's disease.

Understanding Alzheimer's Disease

Understanding Alzheimer's Disease: A Journey Through the Labyrinth

Alzheimer's disease, a progressive and irreversible neurodegenerative condition, casts a long shadow, impacting not just the individual diagnosed but also their loved ones and society as a whole. Understanding this complex disease requires navigating a labyrinth of biological processes, cognitive decline, and emotional challenges. This journey of understanding begins with the hallmarks of the disease – the presence of abnormal proteins called beta-amyloid plaques and tau tangles in the brain. These protein build ups disrupt communication between nerve cells, leading to the characteristic symptoms of Alzheimer's, including memory loss, confusion, and difficulty with daily activities.

As we delve deeper, the stages of the disease unfold, revealing a gradual decline in cognitive function. The early stage may manifest as subtle forgetfulness, while the middle stage brings more pronounced memory loss, personality changes, and difficulty with communication. In the late stage, individuals require complete dependence on caregivers as they lose the ability to perform even basic tasks. However, it's crucial to remember that the progression of Alzheimer's can vary significantly from person to person.

The mystery surrounding the exact causes of Alzheimer's disease continues to intrigue scientists. While age is the biggest risk factor, genetics, environmental factors, and lifestyle choices likely play a role.

Research suggests that chronic inflammation, gut health, and even head injuries may contribute to the development of the disease. Unraveling these intricate connections is essential for unlocking new treatment options and preventative strategies.

Understanding Alzheimer's disease empowers individuals to take control of their situation. Early detection allows for timely treatment and planning for the future. Individuals can learn strategies to manage symptoms, maintain quality of life, and participate in decisions about their care. This knowledge also empowers caregivers – the unsung heroes on the frontlines of this disease. By understanding the stages and challenges faced by individuals with Alzheimer's, caregivers can provide more effective support, manage stress, and navigate their own emotional journey.

The fight against Alzheimer's disease demands a multi-pronged approach. Fueling research and innovation is crucial for identifying new treatment options, exploring preventative strategies, and ultimately, working towards a cure. Understanding the disease empowers researchers to develop targeted therapies, design preventative programs, and advocate for increased funding for research initiatives.

Historical Perspective and Discovery

From Ancient Observations to Modern Diagnosis: A Long Road to Understanding Alzheimer's Disease

The story of Alzheimer's disease is not just a scientific one; it's a saga spanning centuries, reflecting the evolution of our understanding of memory, the brain, and the devastating effects of cognitive decline. This journey begins with ancient observations and progresses to the sophisticated diagnostic tools used today.

Early Glimpses: Memory Loss Through the Ages

References to memory loss and dementia can be traced back to ancient civilizations. Egyptian medical texts from 1,900 BC mention symptoms like forgetfulness and confusion. Greek philosophers like Aristotle pondered the connection between memory and the brain. These early observations, while lacking scientific understanding, hinted at the existence of a condition affecting memory and cognitive function.

The Middle Ages: A Shift in Focus

During the Middle Ages, the focus shifted towards supernatural explanations for dementia. Symptoms were often attributed to demonic possession or witchcraft. This period saw little advancement in understanding the biological basis of memory loss.

The Dawn of Modern Medicine: Unveiling the Brain

The Renaissance ushered in a new era of scientific inquiry. Andreas Vesalius, a 16th-century anatomist, dissected the brain, paving the way for a more scientific understanding of its structure and function. However, the specific causes of memory loss remained a mystery.

Dr. Alois Alzheimer and the First Case: A Turning Point

In 1901, a pivotal moment arrived. Dr. Alois Alzheimer, a German psychiatrist, meticulously documented the case of Auguste D., a woman exhibiting severe memory loss, disorientation, and language difficulties. Upon her death, Dr. Alzheimer examined her brain tissue and discovered abnormal protein deposits, now known as plaques and tangles. This marked the first scientific identification of Alzheimer's disease as a distinct condition.

The 20th Century: Refining the Diagnosis

The 20th century witnessed advancements in diagnosing Alzheimer's disease. In the 1960s, researchers developed criteria for diagnosing the disease based on clinical symptoms and autopsy findings. These criteria, later revised, laid the foundation for the diagnostic tools used today.

Modern Diagnosis: Looking Beyond Symptoms

Today, diagnosing Alzheimer's disease involves a multi-faceted approach. Doctors take into account a patient's medical history, cognitive assessment tests, and brain imaging techniques like MRI and PET scans. These tools allow for earlier and more accurate diagnosis compared to the past.

A Journey Far from Over: The Future of Diagnosis

The quest for an even more definitive diagnosis continues. Researchers are exploring the potential of cerebrospinal fluid analysis and blood tests to identify biomarkers of Alzheimer's disease. These advancements could lead to earlier detection, paving the way for earlier interventions and improved patient outcomes.

From Ancient Whispers to Modern Scans: A Continuous Evolution

The journey from ancient observations of memory loss to the sophisticated diagnostic tools used today highlights the remarkable progress made in understanding Alzheimer's disease. This evolution reflects the tireless efforts of scientists, physicians, and caregivers who have dedicated themselves to unraveling the mysteries of this complex condition. The future holds promise for even more accurate and non-invasive diagnostic methods, empowering us to fight Alzheimer's disease with a greater arsenal of knowledge and tools.

Dr. Alois Alzheimer and the First Case: A Spark that Ignited a Decades-Long Fire

In the annals of medical history, Dr. Alois Alzheimer holds a pivotal position. His meticulous examination of a single patient, Auguste D., in 1901, ignited a firestorm of research that continues to burn brightly over a century later. This section delves into the story of Dr. Alzheimer, his groundbreaking discovery, and the lasting impact it has had on our understanding of Alzheimer's disease.

A Passion for the Brain: The Early Life of Dr. Alzheimer

Born in Bavaria, Germany, in 1864, Alois Alzheimer displayed a keen interest in science and medicine from a young age. He pursued his studies with dedication, earning his medical degree in 1888. His fascination with the brain drew him towards psychiatry, a field still in its early stages of development. In 1888, he began working at the Frankfurt Asylum for Mental and Epileptic Patients, where he would encounter the case that would forever change his career trajectory.

Auguste D.: A Patient with a Puzzling Decline

In 1901, Dr. Alzheimer met Auguste D., a 51-year-old woman exhibiting unusual symptoms. Auguste's memory had begun to deteriorate rapidly. She struggled with basic tasks, became disoriented and suspicious, and her language skills faltered. Intrigued by this atypical presentation of dementia in a relatively young woman, Dr. Alzheimer meticulously documented Auguste's condition over the next five years. He conducted detailed interviews, testing her memory and cognitive function. Despite Auguste's initial resistance, Dr. Alzheimer's persistence in understanding her condition laid the groundwork for a groundbreaking discovery.

Beyond the Symptoms: Unveiling the Hallmarks

Sadly, Auguste's decline continued. In 1906, she passed away. Driven by a desire to understand the biological basis of her symptoms, Dr. Alzheimer requested an autopsy. Examining Auguste's brain tissue under a microscope, he observed a previously unseen pattern. Twisted fibers and abnormal protein deposits, now known as neurofibrillary tangles and beta-amyloid plaques, were present throughout her brain tissue. These hallmarks, as they would later be called, became the cornerstone for identifying Alzheimer's disease as a distinct pathological entity.

A Presentation that Sparked a Revolution:

In 1906, at a psychiatry conference in Tübingen, Dr. Alzheimer presented his findings. He described Auguste's case in detail, highlighting the unusual symptoms and the presence of the previously unseen abnormalities in her brain. This presentation, titled "Presenile Dementia," marked a turning point in our understanding of dementia. While the term "Alzheimer's disease" wouldn't be used until later, Dr. Alzheimer's meticulous observations ignited a firestorm of research into the causes and potential treatments for this devastating condition.

A Legacy of Discovery: The Ripple Effect of Dr. Alzheimer's Work

Dr. Alzheimer's work didn't just identify a new disease; it opened a new chapter in neuroscience. His discovery of the plaques and tangles sparked a wave of research, leading to a deeper understanding of the pathological processes underlying Alzheimer's disease. While Dr. Alzheimer himself died in 1915, unaware of the immense impact of his findings, his legacy continues to inspire scientists and researchers worldwide.

A Century of Progress: Building Upon Dr. Alzheimer's Foundation

Over the past century, Dr. Alzheimer's initial observations have served as a springboard for a vast array of research endeavors. Scientists have explored the role of genetics, environmental factors, and lifestyle choices in the development of Alzheimer's disease. Researchers are actively seeking new treatment options and, ultimately, a cure. The journey started by Dr. Alzheimer with a single patient continues to this day, with scientists and researchers building upon his foundation to combat this devastating disease.

The story of Dr. Alois Alzheimer and Auguste D. is a testament to the power of observation, meticulous documentation, and unwavering curiosity. Their encounter ignited a revolution in our understanding of Alzheimer's disease, paving the way for a future where we can potentially prevent, manage, and ultimately, conquer this memory thief.

Demystifying the Hallmarks: Beyond Plaques and Tangles

While the presence of plaques and tangles remains a defining characteristic of Alzheimer's disease, researchers have delved deeper into understanding their role in the disease process. Advanced imaging techniques have revealed the progression of plaque and tangle formation in the brain, allowing scientists to track their impact on cognitive decline. Furthermore, research suggests that other factors, such as inflammation and a breakdown in communication between neurons, may also contribute to the disease.

Genetics: Unveiling the Code of Risk

The link between genetics and Alzheimer's disease has become increasingly evident. Scientists have identified specific genes associated with an increased risk of developing the disease. While these genes don't guarantee that someone will develop Alzheimer's, they provide valuable clues about an individual's susceptibility. This knowledge has opened doors for exploring personalized medicine approaches, tailoring prevention strategies and treatment options based on an individual's genetic makeup.

Environmental Influences: Shaping Your Risk

Research suggests that environmental factors also play a significant role in the development of Alzheimer's disease. Head injuries, chronic health conditions like diabetes and high blood pressure, exposure to air pollution, and even sleep disturbances have all been linked to an increased risk. Understanding these environmental influences allows individuals to adopt preventive measures and potentially reduce their risk of developing the disease.

Lifestyle Choices: Empowering Your Brain Health

The power of lifestyle choices in protecting brain health is gaining increasing recognition. Research highlights the positive impact of a balanced diet rich in fruits, vegetables, and whole grains. Regular physical activity, mental stimulation through activities like learning a new language or playing chess, and managing stress levels through yoga or meditation can all contribute to cognitive well-being and potentially reduce the risk of Alzheimer's.

Early Detection: A Window of Opportunity

One of the most significant advancements in recent years has been the development of tools for early detection of Alzheimer's disease. Biomarkers, such as specific proteins found in cerebrospinal fluid, and advanced brain imaging techniques allow for earlier diagnosis, enabling individuals to access treatment options and plan for the future while they are still cognitively able to do so. Early detection also paves the way for participation in clinical trials, which are crucial for developing new and more effective treatments.

The Search for a Cure: Exploring New Frontiers

While there is currently no cure for Alzheimer's disease, research is actively exploring new therapeutic avenues. One promising approach focuses on targeting the plaques and tangles in the brain. Scientists are developing drugs to prevent the formation of plaques or to promote their removal, as well as therapies aimed at breaking down tangles. Other research areas include exploring the potential of immunotherapy to harness the body's immune system to attack the plaques and tangles, and investigating the role of inflammation and its potential as a treatment target.

Looking Ahead

The journey to understand Alzheimer's disease has been marked by significant milestones. From Dr. Alzheimer's initial observations to the development of new diagnostic tools and promising therapies, a century of progress has brought us closer to conquering this devastating condition. However, much remains to be unraveled. Continued research holds the key to unlocking the secrets of Alzheimer's disease, paving the way for a future where we can prevent, manage, and ultimately, find a cure for this memory thief. This ongoing exploration demands collaboration between scientists, clinicians, and funding agencies to accelerate the pace of discovery and offer hope to millions affected by Alzheimer's disease.

The fight against Alzheimer's disease is a marathon, not a sprint. Each advancement, each new piece of the puzzle, brings us closer to the ultimate goal. The story of the last century is a testament to human ingenuity and perseverance. By building upon the foundation laid by Dr. Alzheimer and countless others, we can continue to unravel the mysteries of this disease and create a brighter future for individuals and families affected by Alzheimer's disease.

Causes and Risk Factors

Unveiling the Underlying Causes of Alzheimer's Disease

Alzheimer's disease, a thief of memories and destroyer of cognitive function, remains a formidable opponent in the realm of medicine. Unlike some diseases with a single, identifiable cause, Alzheimer's is a complex web woven from multiple threads. This section delves into the multifaceted nature of this disease, exploring the interplay of biological, environmental, and lifestyle factors that contribute to its development.

Genetics: A Loaded Dice Roll

Genetics plays a significant role in the story of Alzheimer's disease. Scientists have identified specific genes, particularly the apolipoprotein E (APOE) gene, that increase a person's susceptibility to the disease. Having a particular variant of the APOE gene, APOE ε4, is a well-established risk factor. However, it's important to understand that genetics is not a deterministic factor. Inheriting a risk gene doesn't guarantee that someone will develop Alzheimer's, and conversely, individuals without these genes can still develop the disease. Genetics influences the odds, but it's not the sole player in this complex game.

Environmental Influences: Beyond Our Genes

The environment in which we live, work, and play also shapes our risk for developing Alzheimer's disease. Head injuries, particularly severe ones, have been linked to an increased risk. Chronic health conditions like diabetes, high blood pressure, and high cholesterol can also contribute to the development of Alzheimer's. Exposure to environmental toxins like air pollution and even sleep disturbances are emerging areas of research as potential risk factors. Understanding these environmental influences allows individuals to adopt preventive measures and potentially mitigate their risk.

The Inflammation and the Brain

Chronic inflammation throughout the body, not just in the brain, is increasingly recognized as a potential player in the development of Alzheimer's disease. This low-grade, persistent inflammation may damage brain cells and contribute to the formation of plaques and tangles. Research suggests that factors like a poor diet, chronic stress, and certain infections may contribute to this inflammatory state. Understanding the link between inflammation and Alzheimer's disease offers promising avenues for potential therapeutic interventions.

The Impact of Lifestyle Choices

The good news is that we are not entirely powerless against Alzheimer's disease. Emerging research highlights the positive impact of healthy lifestyle choices on brain health. A balanced diet rich in fruits, vegetables, and whole grains, combined with regular physical activity, appears to be neuroprotective. Engaging in mentally stimulating activities like learning a new language, playing chess, or doing puzzles may help keep your cognitive faculties sharp. Managing stress through relaxation techniques like yoga or meditation may also contribute to brain health.

A Holistic Approach

The complexity of Alzheimer's disease necessitates a holistic approach that considers the interplay of biological, environmental, and lifestyle factors. Genetics may load the dice, but lifestyle choices and environmental influences can modify the roll. Understanding these intricate connections allows researchers to develop more comprehensive prevention strategies and treatment options. By unraveling the complex web of factors that contribute to Alzheimer's disease, we can move closer to a future where this mind-stealing illness becomes a distant memory.

Genetics: A Predisposition, Not a Guarantee

The specter of Alzheimer's disease can loom large, particularly for those with a family history of the condition. Genetics undoubtedly plays a role in influencing susceptibility, but the narrative surrounding these influences is undergoing a vital shift. This section delves into the evolving understanding of Alzheimer's genetics, highlighting the concept of "predisposition" rather than a deterministic fate.

Beyond the APOE ε4: A Spectrum of Risk

For many years, the apolipoprotein E (APOE) gene, specifically the APOE ε4 variant, held center stage in the discussion of Alzheimer's genetics. Having one or two copies of APOE ε4 increases an individual's risk of developing the disease. However, this doesn't paint the whole picture. Firstly, a significant portion of people with APOE ε4 never develop Alzheimer's. Secondly, numerous other genes have been identified as potential risk factors, each with varying degrees of influence. This emerging understanding highlights the complex interplay of genetics in Alzheimer's, moving away from a single-gene narrative.

Epigenetics

Epigenetics, the field studying how genes are expressed, adds another layer of complexity. Imagine genes as instructions for building a house. Epigenetics acts like a dimmer switch, regulating how loudly those instructions are "heard." Environmental factors like diet, stress, and lifestyle choices can influence epigenetic modifications, turning genes on or off. This suggests that even individuals with a genetic predisposition may be able to modulate their risk through healthy lifestyle choices.

The Power of Resilience Genes

The human genome isn't solely populated by risk factors. An exciting area of research focuses on "resilience genes" that may offer protection against Alzheimer's disease. These genes, while less studied than risk factors, may act as a buffer, mitigating the negative effects of other genes or environmental factors. Identifying and understanding these resilience genes holds immense potential for developing personalized preventive strategies.

Polygenic Risk Scores

The field of Alzheimer's genetics is moving towards a more nuanced approach. Researchers are developing "polygenic risk scores" that consider the combined impact of multiple genes, not just the APOE ε4 variant. These scores, while still under development, offer a more holistic picture of an individual's genetic susceptibility. However, it's crucial to remember that these scores are not a crystal ball; they predict risk, not destiny.

Beyond Genes

The focus on genetics shouldn't overshadow the importance of other factors in Alzheimer's disease. Environmental influences, lifestyle choices, and overall health all play a significant role. A healthy diet, regular exercise, and managing stress levels can potentially mitigate the impact of genetic risk factors. Furthermore, a supportive social network and a sense of purpose in life can contribute to cognitive resilience.

From Passive to Active

Understanding the role of genetics in Alzheimer's disease empowers individuals to take a more active role in their health. It's not about passively waiting for a disease to strike; it's about embracing a proactive approach. By understanding their genetic predisposition, individuals can work with healthcare professionals to create personalized plans that emphasize healthy lifestyle choices and potentially mitigate their risk. This shift in perspective empowers individuals to move from feeling like victims of their genes to proactive participants in their brain health.

The Future of Genetics in Alzheimer's Research

The field of Alzheimer's genetics is rapidly evolving. As researchers delve deeper into the complex interplay of genes, the environment, and lifestyle, new avenues for prevention and treatment will emerge.

Identifying resilience genes, developing more accurate polygenic risk scores, and exploring the role of epigenetics all hold immense promise. The story of Alzheimer's genetics is no longer one of deterministic fate; it's a narrative of empowerment, offering a beacon of hope in the fight against this debilitating disease.

Environmental Exposures and the Multi-Hit Hypothesis of Alzheimer's Disease

While the precise etiology of Alzheimer's disease (AD) remains elusive, a growing body of research suggests a multi-hit hypothesis. This model posits that AD arises from a complex interplay between genetic susceptibility and environmental exposures that trigger a cascade of neurodegenerative events. This section delves into the technical aspects of how environmental factors may contribute to the development of AD.

Head Injuries: A Disruption of Cellular Homeostasis

Head injuries, particularly severe ones like traumatic brain injuries (TBIs), are a well-established risk factor for AD. The mechanical forces exerted during a TBI can lead to a multitude of cellular disruptions. Axonal shearing, the tearing of nerve fibers, disrupts communication between brain cells. Blood-brain barrier (BBB) dysfunction, a breakdown of the tight junctions that protect the brain from harmful substances in the bloodstream, can lead to chronic neuroinflammation. Furthermore, TBI can trigger the accumulation of abnormal protein aggregates, including tau and amyloid-beta, which are hallmarks of AD pathology.

Chronic Health Conditions: A Double-Edged Sword

Several chronic health conditions are associated with an increased risk of AD. Diabetes mellitus type 2 (T2DM) disrupts insulin signaling pathways crucial for brain function and can lead to chronic inflammation, both of which contribute to neurodegeneration. Hypertension, or high blood pressure, can damage the delicate vasculature of the brain, leading to reduced blood flow and oxygen supply to brain cells. Chronic hyperlipidemia, elevated levels of cholesterol and other fats in the blood, may contribute to the formation of amyloid plaques in the brain. Interestingly, these chronic conditions often co-occur, creating a synergistic effect on AD risk.

The Insidious Threat of Environmental Toxins

Exposure to environmental toxins may also play a role in the development of AD. Air pollution, particularly fine particulate matter (PM2.5), has been linked to an increased risk. These microscopic particles can breach the BBB and trigger neuroinflammation. Heavy metals like lead and aluminum have also been implicated in AD, although the exact mechanisms are still under investigation. Pesticides and other environmental contaminants may also contribute to neurodegeneration, but further research is needed to solidify these connections.

The Microbiome Connection: A Gut Feeling About Brain Health

The gut microbiome, the vast community of microorganisms residing in our intestines, is increasingly recognized as a potential player in AD. Dysbiosis, an imbalance in the gut microbiome composition, has been linked to chronic inflammation and impaired blood-brain barrier function. These disruptions may contribute to the development of AD pathology. Furthermore, the gut microbiome may influence the production of amyloid-beta and tau proteins, further solidifying the potential link between gut health and brain health.

Cellular Stress Pathways: A Common Denominator

Many environmental exposures, from head injuries to chronic health conditions and environmental toxins, converge on a common pathway – cellular stress. These stressors can activate the unfolded protein response (UPR), a cellular mechanism designed to deal with misfolded proteins. However, chronic stress can overwhelm the UPR, leading to the accumulation of misfolded proteins like tau and amyloid-beta, a hallmark of AD. Furthermore, chronic stress can trigger neuroinflammation, further exacerbating neurodegeneration.

Navigating the Environmental Landscape: Mitigation Strategies

Understanding the environmental factors that contribute to AD risk empowers individuals to adopt preventive measures. Maintaining good cardiovascular health through diet and exercise can mitigate the risk associated with conditions like T2DM and hypertension. Wearing protective gear during activities that increase the risk of head injuries, such as contact sports, can help reduce TBI risk. Minimizing exposure to air pollution by limiting time outdoors on high smog days and choosing residences in areas with lower air pollution levels may be beneficial. While completely eliminating environmental risk factors may not be possible, adopting a proactive approach can potentially lower overall risk.

The Future of Environmental Research in AD

Research into the environmental factors that contribute to AD is ongoing. Investigating the precise mechanisms by which these exposures trigger neurodegeneration will be crucial for developing targeted interventions. Furthermore, exploring potential interactions between genetic predisposition and environmental risk factors holds promise for personalized risk assessment and prevention strategies. By unraveling the intricate web of environmental influences, we can refine the multi-hit hypothesis and pave the way for a more comprehensive understanding of AD.

Optimizing Neuroprotective Pathways Through Lifestyle Choices

Alzheimer's disease (AD) presents a formidable challenge, marked by progressive cognitive decline and neurodegeneration. While a definitive cure remains elusive, mounting evidence suggests that lifestyle choices can significantly impact brain health and potentially reduce AD risk. This section delves into the technical aspects of how specific lifestyle modifications activate neuroprotective pathways, bolstering cognitive resilience.

Dietary Choices: Fueling the Brain for Optimal Performance

The brain, a metabolic powerhouse, is highly dependent on a steady supply of nutrients. A balanced diet rich in fruits, vegetables, and whole grains provides essential vitamins, minerals, and antioxidants that support neuronal function and protect against oxidative stress. Omega-3 fatty acids, found in oily fish, play a crucial role in maintaining neuronal membranes and promoting synaptogenesis, the formation of new synapses, which is critical for learning and memory. Conversely, diets high in saturated fats, refined carbohydrates, and added sugars have been linked to cognitive decline and increased AD risk. These dietary patterns promote chronic inflammation, impair insulin signaling, and contribute to the development of insulin resistance, which can negatively impact brain function.

Physical Activity: A Symphony of Neuroprotective Effects

Regular physical activity emerges as a potent neuroprotective strategy. Exercise promotes brain-derived neurotrophic factor (BDNF) production. BDNF acts like a fertilizer for the brain, fostering the growth and survival of neurons, enhancing synaptic plasticity, and promoting overall cognitive function. Physical activity also increases cerebral blood flow, delivering essential oxygen and nutrients to brain cells. Furthermore, exercise triggers the release of endorphins, which have mood-boosting and neuroprotective effects. The benefits extend beyond the brain; exercise improves cardiovascular health, reduces inflammation, and promotes better sleep, all of which contribute to cognitive well-being.

Cognitive Engagement: Keeping the Neural Networks Firing

The brain thrives on stimulation. Engaging in mentally stimulating activities like learning a new language, playing chess, or solving puzzles strengthens existing neural connections and promotes the formation of new ones. This cognitive exercise keeps the brain's "wiring" robust and adaptable, potentially delaying cognitive decline. Furthermore, mentally stimulating activities can enhance cognitive reserve, the brain's ability to compensate for age-related changes or neuropathological processes. By challenging the brain to adapt and learn, individuals can potentially build up a cognitive "buffer" against neurodegenerative diseases like AD.

Sleep: A Time for Cellular Housekeeping

Sleep plays a vital role in brain health and cognitive function. During deep sleep, the brain engages in a process called glymphatic clearance, where waste products like amyloid-beta, a hallmark of AD pathology, are cleared from the brain tissue. Chronic sleep deprivation disrupts this clearance process, potentially leading to the accumulation of amyloid-beta and its associated neurodegenerative effects. Furthermore, sleep deprivation impairs cognitive function, memory consolidation, and emotional regulation. Aiming for 7-8 hours of quality sleep each night is crucial for optimal brain health and the clearance of potentially neurotoxic waste products.

Stress Management: Calming the Inflammatory Cascade

Chronic stress can have a detrimental impact on brain health. When stressed, the body releases stress hormones like cortisol, which can damage neurons and impair hippocampal function, a brain region critical for memory. Chronic stress also triggers a pro-inflammatory cascade, contributing to neurodegeneration. Conversely, techniques like mindfulness meditation, yoga, and deep breathing activate the parasympathetic nervous system, promoting relaxation and reducing stress hormone levels. These practices also dampen the inflammatory response, creating a neuroprotective environment for the brain.

The Synergy of Lifestyle Factors: A Multifaceted Approach

The impact of lifestyle choices on brain health is not a single, isolated effect; it's a symphony of interconnected benefits. A diet rich in brain-healthy nutrients combined with regular physical activity, cognitive stimulation, quality sleep, and effective stress management strategies work synergistically to create a neuroprotective environment. This multifaceted approach not only promotes overall well-being but also potentially reduces the risk of developing AD.

Precision Lifestyle Medicine: Tailoring Strategies for Individual Needs

The field of precision lifestyle medicine holds immense promise for the future of brain health and AD prevention. By considering an individual's genetic makeup, gut microbiome composition, and overall health status, personalized lifestyle recommendations can be tailored to maximize neuroprotective benefits. This approach recognizes that there is no "one-size-fits-all" strategy and that optimizing brain health requires a customized approach.

Common Symptoms and Manifestations

Alzheimer's disease (AD) is a neurodegenerative disorder characterized by a progressive decline in cognitive function. Unlike the occasional forgetfulness we all experience, AD symptoms steadily worsen, disrupting daily life and independence. This section delves into the technical aspects of the most common symptoms and manifestations of AD, providing a deeper understanding of how the disease disrupts various cognitive domains.

Episodic Memory: The Erosion of the Autobiographical Self

Episodic memory, the cornerstone of our autobiographical self, allows us to encode, store, and retrieve personal experiences. It's the memory that allows us to recall details from our birthday party last year or that heartwarming conversation with a loved one. AD disrupts this system at its core. The hallmark neuropathology – amyloid plaques and neurofibrillary tangles – disrupts the hippocampus, a seahorse-shaped structure crucial for memory consolidation. Early symptoms often manifest as forgetting recently learned information, misplaced items, or difficulty recalling details from past experiences. As the disease progresses, these episodic memory deficits become more pronounced. Individuals may struggle to remember recent events, conversations, or appointments. In severe cases, they may forget significant life events or even struggle to recognize themselves in the mirror.

Executive Function: The Conductor Loses Control of the Orchestra

Executive function encompasses a set of higher-order cognitive skills that orchestrate our daily lives. Planning, organizing, multitasking, problem-solving, and decision-making all fall under this umbrella. The prefrontal cortex, a region heavily implicated in AD pathology, plays a central role in executive function. As the disease progresses, the disruption in these neural circuits manifests as difficulties planning and organizing tasks. Individuals may struggle to follow multi-step instructions, create grocery lists, or manage finances. Decision-making becomes impaired, leading to poor choices or impulsivity. Adapting to new situations and problem-solving become increasingly challenging. These impairments significantly impact daily functioning and independence, often requiring assistance with managing finances, medications, and household chores.

Language: A Breakdown in Communication

Language is a complex tapestry woven from various cognitive threads. Aphasia, a language disorder characterized by difficulties with speaking, understanding spoken language, reading, and writing, can be a prominent symptom in some individuals with AD. The specific language impairments depend on the location of the neurodegeneration. Anomia, the frustrating inability to find the right word, is a common early symptom. Individuals may struggle to name familiar objects, describe events, or participate in conversations. Agrammatism, where sentences lack proper grammar and structure, can also occur. These language impairments can lead to profound communication difficulties, social isolation, and frustration for both the individual and their caregivers.

Visuospatial Dysfunction: Losing Sight of the Bigger Picture

Visuospatial function encompasses our ability to perceive, process, and interact with the spatial environment. While not a core feature of AD, visuospatial dysfunction can be a significant challenge for some individuals. Difficulties with interpreting visual information, navigating unfamiliar environments, judging distances, or performing tasks requiring spatial awareness can arise. These impairments can lead to difficulties driving, navigating through crowds, or even completing simple tasks like pouring liquids.

Beyond Cognition: The Emotional Toll of AD

While cognitive decline is a hallmark feature, AD also manifests through a range of non-cognitive symptoms collectively termed Behavioral and Psychological Symptoms of Dementia (BPSD). Depression, anxiety, apathy, agitation, and sleep disturbances are common BPSD manifestations. These symptoms can arise from the underlying neurodegeneration itself, medication side effects, or the frustration associated with cognitive decline. Furthermore, the disruption in communication and social interaction can lead to feelings of isolation and loneliness, further exacerbating BPSD. Effective management of BPSD is crucial for improving quality of life for individuals with AD and their caregivers.

A Spectrum of Manifestations: A Heterogeneous Disease

It's important to remember that AD is a heterogeneous disease, with the presentation and rate of progression varying significantly from person to person. Some individuals may experience memory decline as the predominant symptom, while others may struggle more with language or visuospatial difficulties. The rate of progression can also differ, with some individuals experiencing a rapid decline and others progressing more slowly. Early diagnosis and a comprehensive understanding of the specific symptoms and manifestations are crucial for tailoring treatment plans and maximizing quality of life for individuals living with AD.

Impairments in Episodic Memory

Episodic memory, the cornerstone of our autobiographical self, allows us to encode, store, and retrieve vivid details of personal experiences. It's the memory that lets you recount that delicious meal you had with friends last week, the details of your recent vacation, or the heartwarming conversation with a loved one. In Alzheimer's disease (AD), episodic memory is one of the earliest and most prominent cognitive domains to be affected. This section delves into the technical aspects of how the neuropathology of AD disrupts the intricate machinery of episodic memory, leading to the erosion of recent experiences.

The Hippocampus: A Vulnerable Hub for Memory Consolidation

The hippocampus, a seahorse-shaped structure nestled deep within the temporal lobe, plays a central role in episodic memory. This critical brain region acts as a processing center, responsible for encoding new information into long-term memories. It facilitates the consolidation process, transforming fleeting experiences into lasting memories. In AD, the hallmark neuropathology – the accumulation of amyloid-beta plaques and neurofibrillary tangles – disrupts the delicate machinery of the hippocampus. Amyloid-beta plaques, deposits of protein fragments, disrupt communication between neurons by interfering with neurotransmitters like glutamate, essential for memory formation. Neurofibrillary tangles, formed by abnormal tau protein aggregates, damage the internal structure of neurons, further impairing their ability to function properly. This cumulative assault on the hippocampus weakens its ability to encode and consolidate new information, leading to the characteristic memory decline observed in AD.

Synaptic Dysfunction: A Breakdown in Communication Highways

Memories are formed through the strengthening of connections, or synapses, between neurons. During the process of encoding new information, the hippocampus orchestrates a complex cascade of events that strengthens these synaptic connections. However, in AD, the neurodegenerative processes disrupt this delicate dance. The buildup of amyloid-beta plaques and neurofibrillary tangles hinders the release of neurotransmitters, essential for communication between neurons. Furthermore, these pathological processes can lead to the loss of dendritic spines, tiny protrusions on neurons that increase their surface area and enhance communication efficiency. This cumulative effect weakens existing synaptic connections and hinders the formation of new ones, leading to difficulties forming new memories and impaired retrieval of existing ones.

Theta Wave Disruption: The Orchestra Loses its Rhythm

Electrophysiological recordings of the brain reveal a characteristic pattern of brain waves during memory encoding and retrieval. Theta waves, rhythmic brain activity in the 4-8 Hz range, are particularly important for episodic memory function. In individuals with AD, theta wave activity becomes disrupted and disorganized. This dysrhythmia reflects the dysfunction within the hippocampal network, further hindering the efficient processing and consolidation of new information.

A Cascade of Failures: From Encoding Deficits to Retrieval Impairments

The impairments in episodic memory in AD are not isolated events. The disruption in the hippocampus due to the underlying neuropathology creates a cascade of failures. Difficulties with encoding new information lead to a decline in the formation of new memories. As the disease progresses, the retrieval of existing memories also becomes impaired. The weakened synaptic connections and the disrupted communication within the hippocampal network make it increasingly challenging to access and recall stored memories. Initially, individuals may forget recent events or struggle to recall specific details. In the later stages of AD, even remote memories may become inaccessible, leading to a profound loss of personal history and a sense of self.

Understanding the Mechanisms: Paving the Way for Future Interventions

Delving into the technical aspects of how AD disrupts episodic memory is crucial not only for understanding the symptoms but also for paving the way for future interventions. By pinpointing the specific cellular and molecular mechanisms involved, researchers can develop targeted therapies aimed at protecting the hippocampus, enhancing synaptic function, and promoting memory consolidation. Furthermore, a deeper understanding of these processes can guide the development of early diagnostic tools and interventions aimed at slowing the progression of memory decline in AD.

Executive Function

Executive function, the maestro of our cognitive orchestra, conducts a complex symphony of higher-order skills crucial for navigating daily life. It encompasses planning, organizing, multitasking, problem-solving, decision-making, and cognitive flexibility. In Alzheimer's disease (AD), the gradual neurodegeneration disrupts this intricate network, turning the once-smooth performance into a cacophony of cognitive challenges. This section delves into the technical aspects of how AD disrupts the neural underpinnings of executive function, leading to a decline in independence and daily living skills.

The Prefrontal Cortex: The Command Center Under Siege

The prefrontal cortex (PFC), the brain region nestled behind the forehead, plays a central role in executive function. It acts as the maestro, coordinating the activity of various brain regions responsible for memory retrieval, planning, inhibition, and goal-directed behavior. In AD, the hallmark neuropathology, including amyloid-beta plaques and neurofibrillary tangles, heavily targets the PFC. These pathological hallmarks disrupt the delicate communication between neurons, impairing the PFC's ability to effectively orchestrate cognitive processes. Furthermore, the loss of neurons within the PFC due to neurodegeneration further weakens its functionality. This assault on the PFC disrupts the delicate balance between different cognitive processes, leading to the characteristic executive dysfunction observed in AD.

Disrupted Working Memory

Working memory, a cognitive subcomponent of executive function, acts as the temporary holding space for information and facilitates its manipulation during complex tasks. It's akin to the sheet music the maestro holds while conducting – vital for keeping track of the musical flow. In AD, the disruption in the PFC due to neurodegeneration impairs working memory function. Individuals may struggle to retain multi-step instructions, forget midway through completing a task, or lose track of objects they placed down moments ago. These working memory deficits significantly impact the ability to plan and sequence complex activities, leading to difficulties with tasks such as cooking a meal, following a recipe, or balancing a checkbook.

Decision-Making: From Calculated Choices to Impulsive Blunders

Effective decision-making requires weighing options, evaluating risks and rewards, and selecting the most appropriate course of action. The PFC plays a critical role in this process. In AD, the disruption in the

PFC impairs the ability to critically assess situations, leading to poor choices and impulsive behaviors. Individuals may make financially risky decisions, struggle to weigh the consequences of their actions, or become easily influenced by others. These impaired decision-making abilities can have significant consequences for daily life, jeopardizing financial security and safety.

Cognitive Flexibility: Difficulty Adapting to the Changing Tempo

Cognitive flexibility refers to the ability to adapt our thoughts and behaviors in response to changing demands. Imagine the orchestra needing to adjust its tempo or key unexpectedly. In a healthy brain, the PFC facilitates this cognitive flexibility, allowing us to adjust plans or approaches when encountering unforeseen situations. In AD, the disrupted PFC function leads to difficulties adapting to new situations. Individuals may struggle to switch tasks mid-stream, become fixated on routines, or have difficulty implementing new strategies to solve problems. This inflexibility can lead to frustration and difficulty navigating the ever-changing demands of daily life.

A Cascade of Consequences: From Cognitive Decline to Functional Impairment

The impairments in executive function in AD have a profound impact on daily living. Individuals may struggle to manage finances, plan meals, take medications on schedule, or follow schedules. The inability to make sound decisions can lead to financial exploitation or unsafe situations. As the disease progresses, the need for assistance with daily activities increases, significantly impacting independence and quality of life.

Exploring Neuroprotective Strategies

Understanding the technical underpinnings of how AD disrupts executive function is crucial not only for diagnosis but also for identifying potential therapeutic approaches. Research efforts are focused on neuroprotective strategies that can protect the PFC from neurodegeneration, enhance neural communication, and support cognitive function. Furthermore, cognitive rehabilitation techniques can be employed to help individuals with AD develop compensatory strategies to work around their executive function challenges.

Language: A Breakdown in Communication - A Neurodegenerative side to Alzheimer's Disease

Language, the cornerstone of human interaction, allows us to express thoughts, share experiences, and build meaningful connections. In Alzheimer's disease (AD), the delicate machinery of language unravels, leading to a progressive decline in communication abilities. This section delves into the intricate neurological underpinnings of language and explores how AD disrupts this symphony of cognitive processes, resulting in a breakdown in communication.

The Neural Orchestra of Language: A Delicate Balance of Regions

Language processing is not a singular act but a complex symphony orchestrated by a network of brain regions. The dominant hemisphere, typically the left hemisphere, plays a leading role. Broca's area, located in the frontal lobe, is responsible for speech production – the act of formulating thoughts into spoken words. Wernicke's area, situated in the temporal lobe, is crucial for language comprehension – the ability to understand spoken language. The arcuate fasciculus, a white matter pathway, serves as the vital bridge connecting these regions, enabling the seamless flow of information between them. In addition to these core areas, a network of interconnected regions contributes to various aspects of language, including fluency, grammar, and semantic processing (understanding word meaning).

The Insidious Grip of AD: Disrupting the Neural Symphony

The hallmark neuropathology of AD, amyloid-beta plaques and neurofibrillary tangles, disrupts the delicate balance within the language network. These pathological hallmarks disrupt communication between neurons, hindering the flow of information within and between brain regions. Furthermore, the neurodegeneration characteristic of AD leads to a progressive loss of neurons, particularly in vulnerable regions like Broca's and Wernicke's areas. This cumulative assault on the neural architecture of language translates into a breakdown in communication abilities observed in individuals with AD.

Aphasia

Aphasia, a language disorder characterized by difficulties with speaking, understanding spoken language, reading, and writing, is a prominent manifestation of language breakdown in AD. The specific type of aphasia depends on the location and severity of the neurodegeneration.

Anomia

One of the earliest language symptoms in AD, anomia manifests as the frustrating inability to find the right word. Individuals may struggle to name familiar objects, describe events, or participate in conversations, leading to a sense of frustration and social isolation.

Agrammatism: This form of aphasia affects sentence structure and grammar. Individuals with agrammatism may speak in short, telegraphic phrases lacking proper grammatical structure, making their speech difficult to understand.

Wernicke's aphasia: Damage to Wernicke's area can lead to Wernicke's aphasia, characterized by difficulties understanding spoken language. Individuals may struggle to follow conversations, misinterpret what is being said, or have difficulty forming coherent responses.

Beyond Words: A Breakdown in Non-Verbal Communication

Language extends beyond spoken words. Prosody, the rhythm, intonation, and emotional tone of speech, is crucial for conveying meaning and intent. In AD, the disruption in neural networks responsible for emotional processing can lead to impairments in prosody. Individuals may speak in a flat monotone, making their speech sound emotionless or robotic. Furthermore, nonverbal communication through facial expressions and gestures may also be affected, hindering the ability to effectively convey emotions and ideas.

The language impairments in AD vary significantly from person to person. Some individuals may experience predominantly anomia, while others may struggle more with comprehension or fluency. The rate of progression can also differ, with some individuals experiencing a rapid decline in language abilities and others showing a more gradual decline.

The Emotional Toll of Language Breakdown

The breakdown in communication in AD can be incredibly isolating and frustrating for both the individual and their caregivers. The inability to express oneself clearly or understand what others are saying can lead to feelings of loneliness, depression, and anxiety. Furthermore, the frustration associated with language difficulties can manifest as behavioral outbursts or agitation.

Visuospatial Dysfunction: A Descent into Disorientation in Alzheimer's Disease

Visuospatial function, the intricate dance between vision and spatial cognition, allows us to navigate the world with confidence. It encompasses a constellation of abilities – interpreting visual information, perceiving depth and distance, mentally manipulating objects in space, and coordinating our movements through our environment. While not a defining feature of Alzheimer's disease (AD), visuospatial dysfunction can be a significant and under-recognized challenge for some individuals, impacting daily life and independence. This section delves into the technical underpinnings of visuospatial processing and explores how AD disrupts these systems, leading to a descent into disorientation.

The Neural Orchestra of Visuospatial Processing: A Multi-Sensory Collaboration

Visuospatial processing is not a singular act but a complex symphony orchestrated by a network of interconnected brain regions. The primary visual cortex, located in the occipital lobe, receives visual information from the eyes. This information is then relayed to various other brain regions for further processing. The parietal lobe plays a crucial role in integrating visual information with spatial cues, allowing us to perceive depth, judge distances, and manipulate objects in space. The temporal lobe contributes to visual memory and object recognition. Furthermore, the frontal lobe is essential for spatial planning and coordinating our movements through the environment. A seamless flow of information between these regions and integration with other sensory inputs like touch and proprioception (body awareness) is crucial for robust visuospatial function.

The Insidious Grip of AD: Disrupting the Spatial Awareness

The hallmark neuropathology of AD, amyloid-beta plaques and neurofibrillary tangles, can disrupt the delicate balance within the visuospatial network in several ways:

Disrupted Information Processing: The accumulation of these pathological hallmarks disrupts communication between neurons within and between brain regions involved in visuospatial processing. This hinders the seamless flow of visual information, making it difficult to interpret complex visual scenes or integrate spatial cues.

Neuronal Loss: In AD, the neurodegenerative process leads to a progressive loss of neurons, including those within the parietal and temporal lobes critical for spatial processing and object recognition. This loss further weakens the neural architecture underpinning visuospatial function.

Disruption of White Matter Tracts: White matter pathways serve as the information highways connecting different brain regions. In AD, the disruption of white matter integrity can hinder the efficient communication between areas crucial for visuospatial processing.

Manifestations of Visuospatial Dysfunction: From Getting Lost to Difficulty Completing Tasks

The disruption of the visuospatial network in AD can manifest in various ways:

Visuospatial Agnosia: Difficulty recognizing familiar objects despite intact vision. Individuals may struggle to identify objects in everyday settings or perceive depth and three-dimensionality.

Topographical Disorientation: Difficulties navigating familiar environments, getting lost in previously known places, or struggling with route planning. This can be particularly concerning for individuals with AD who may wander and become disoriented.

Constructional Apraxia: Inability to copy simple drawings or assemble objects from components. This may arise due to difficulties with spatial planning and coordinating movements necessary for these tasks.

Hemispatial Neglect: A deficit in attending to one side of the visual field, typically the left side. This can lead to difficulties driving, eating, or dressing as individuals may neglect one side of their body.

Beyond the Visual: The Impact on Daily Life

Visuospatial dysfunction in AD can significantly impact daily activities and independence. Difficulties judging distances can lead to falls or difficulty pouring liquids. Impairments in spatial planning and navigation can hinder the ability to complete everyday tasks like dressing, cooking, or managing finances. Furthermore, the frustration and anxiety associated with getting lost or disoriented can contribute to behavioral changes and social withdrawal.

It's important to remember that AD is a heterogeneous disease, with the severity and presentation of visuospatial dysfunction varying significantly among individuals. Some people with AD may experience minimal visuospatial difficulties throughout the course of the disease, while others may display prominent challenges early on. The presence and severity of visuospatial dysfunction can also influence the overall functional decline and require tailored support strategies.

Early diagnosis: Visuospatial testing can be a valuable tool for identifying early signs of AD, particularly in individuals presenting with atypical symptoms.

Development of targeted interventions: By pinpointing the specific brain regions and pathways affected, research efforts can be directed towards developing therapies aimed at improving visuospatial function or enhancing compensatory strategies.

Individualized care plans: Understanding the specific visuospatial challenges faced by an individual with AD allows caregivers

Diagnosis and Treatment

Diagnosing Alzheimer's disease (AD) can be a complex process, often requiring a multi-pronged approach that incorporates various diagnostic tools. This section delves into the different procedures and tests used to evaluate for AD, providing a roadmap for navigating the diagnostic journey.

Diagnostic procedures and tests for Alzheimer's Disease

An accurate diagnosis of Alzheimer's disease (AD) is crucial for initiating appropriate treatment and planning for future care. The clinical evaluation serves as the cornerstone of the diagnostic process, laying the groundwork for further investigations. This section delves into the various components of a comprehensive clinical evaluation and explores how it helps build a strong foundation for diagnosing AD.

A Detailed History: Unveiling the Pieces of the Puzzle

The clinical evaluation begins with a detailed medical and family history. The physician will inquire about:

Current symptoms: A thorough understanding of the individual's cognitive decline, including the onset, progression, and specific memory difficulties, is crucial. Family members or caregivers can be valuable sources of information in this regard.

Past medical history: Certain medical conditions, such as head injury, stroke, or thyroid problems, can sometimes mimic symptoms of AD. A comprehensive medical history helps identify these potential contributors.

Medications: Some medications can cause cognitive side effects that may be mistaken for AD. The physician will review the current medication regimen to rule out this possibility.

Family history: A family history of dementia, particularly AD, increases the risk of developing the disease. Identifying any family members with cognitive decline can provide valuable information.

Mental Status Examination: Assessing Cognitive Function at the Bedside

The mental status examination (MSE) is a brief, standardized assessment tool used to evaluate an individual's cognitive state at the time of the evaluation. The MSE typically covers various domains, including:

Orientation: This assesses awareness of time, place, and person. In AD, individuals may become disoriented to time or place, particularly in later stages.

Attention and concentration: The physician may ask the individual to perform simple tasks like repeating numbers or following instructions to assess their ability to focus and maintain attention.

Memory: Short-term and long-term memory functions are evaluated. The physician may ask the individual to recall recent events or long-term memories from their past to identify any memory deficits.

Language: The MSE assesses an individual's ability to express themselves clearly, understand spoken language, and follow commands. Difficulties with word-finding or sentence structure may indicate language problems associated with AD.

Executive function: Simple tasks that require planning or problem-solving skills may be used to assess executive function, which can be impaired in AD.

Neurological Examination: Looking for Signs of Underlying Pathology

The neurological examination assesses the functioning of the nervous system. While not specific for AD, some abnormalities may provide clues about the underlying pathology. The examination may include:

Motor function: Checking for tremors, coordination issues, or weakness can help rule out other neurological conditions that may mimic AD symptoms.

Reflexes: Abnormal reflexes can sometimes indicate damage to the nervous system.

Sensory function: Vision and hearing difficulties can sometimes contribute to cognitive decline, and assessing these functions is important.

Building the Clinical Picture: Integrating the Pieces

The information gathered from the detailed medical and family history, mental status examination, and neurological examination is meticulously integrated to create a comprehensive clinical picture. The physician will consider factors such as the age of onset, the pattern of cognitive decline, the presence of specific symptoms, and the absence of other potential explanations for the cognitive decline.

Limitations of the Clinical Evaluation

While the clinical evaluation is a crucial first step, it has limitations. The symptoms of AD can sometimes overlap with other forms of dementia, making a definitive diagnosis based solely on clinical presentation challenging. Furthermore, the clinical evaluation cannot visualize the underlying neuropathology of AD in the brain.

The Foundation for Further Investigation: Paving the Way for a Definitive Diagnosis

Despite these limitations, the detailed information gleaned from the clinical evaluation sets the stage for further investigations. Based on the findings, the physician may recommend additional tests, such as neuropsychological assessments, brain imaging studies, or biomarker testing, to reach a more definitive diagnosis of AD. The clinical evaluation serves as a vital roadmap, guiding the diagnostic journey and ensuring that the appropriate tools are employed for accurate diagnosis of Alzheimer's disease.

Neuropsychological Assessment: Gauging Cognitive Function in Alzheimer's Disease

The clinical evaluation provides a valuable snapshot of an individual's cognitive state, but for a more in-depth exploration of cognitive function in suspected Alzheimer's disease (AD), a neuropsychological assessment becomes crucial. This specialized evaluation, conducted by a neuropsychologist, delves deeper into various cognitive domains, providing a comprehensive picture of strengths and weaknesses.

A Battery of Tests: Unveiling the Cognitive Landscape

A neuropsychological assessment for AD typically employs a battery of standardized tests that evaluate various cognitive domains:

Memory: A range of tests assess different aspects of memory function. Immediate and delayed recall tasks evaluate short-term and long-term memory, respectively. Verbal and visual memory domains are often explored separately, as some individuals may exhibit greater difficulty with one type of memory over the other. Recognition tasks assess the ability to identify previously encountered information.

Attention and Concentration: Tests measuring sustained attention and the ability to filter out distractions are used. Individuals with AD may struggle to maintain focus for prolonged periods or become easily sidetracked by environmental stimuli.

Language: Fluency, comprehension, and naming abilities are evaluated. Word-finding difficulties, problems with sentence structure, or difficulty understanding complex language may be indicative of language impairments associated with AD.

Executive Function: Tasks requiring planning, organizing, problem-solving, and decision-making are employed. Difficulties with these skills can significantly impact daily living and are often prominent in AD.

Visuospatial Function: The ability to perceive, process, and interact with spatial information is assessed. Individuals with AD may exhibit difficulties with tasks like copying drawings, navigating unfamiliar environments, or judging distances.

Beyond Scores: Interpreting the Cognitive Profile

The raw scores obtained on individual tests are not the sole focus of a neuropsychological assessment. The neuropsychologist meticulously analyzes the pattern of performance across different cognitive domains, looking for specific weaknesses that may point towards AD. Here are some key aspects considered:

Discrepancies: A significant disparity in performance between different cognitive domains can be a red flag for AD. For example, profound memory deficits with relatively preserved language skills may suggest AD compared to a more even decline across domains.

Comparison to Normative Data: Test scores are compared to established norms for age and education to determine if performance falls within the expected range. Significant deviations from expected performance can indicate cognitive impairment.

Changes over Time: When possible, comparing current test results to prior assessments can be particularly informative. A decline in performance on previously mastered tasks can be a strong indicator of progressive cognitive decline.

Advantages of Neuropsychological Assessment

Neuropsychological assessments offer several advantages in the diagnostic workup of AD:

Comprehensive Evaluation: They provide a detailed picture of cognitive strengths and weaknesses, offering a more nuanced understanding of the individual's cognitive profile.

Differential Diagnosis: The specific pattern of cognitive decline can help differentiate AD from other forms of dementia that may have different underlying pathologies.

Monitoring Progression: Repeated assessments over time can track the progression of cognitive decline and guide treatment decisions.

Limitations of Neuropsychological Assessment

While valuable, neuropsychological assessments also have limitations:

Time-Consuming: These assessments can be lengthy, requiring significant time and effort from both the patient and the neuropsychologist.

Practice Effects: Repeated exposure to similar tests can lead to improved performance over time, which may not accurately reflect true cognitive abilities.

Cultural and Educational Bias: Some standardized tests may be biased towards specific cultural backgrounds or educational levels.

A Crucial Piece in the Diagnostic Puzzle

Current treatment options and medications

While there is currently no cure for Alzheimer's disease (AD), treatment options are available to manage symptoms, improve quality of life, and potentially slow the progression of the disease. This section explores the different categories of medications and treatment approaches currently used in AD management.

Medications for Managing Cognitive Symptoms in Alzheimer's Disease: A Modulatory Approach

Alzheimer's disease (AD) is a progressive neurodegenerative disorder characterized by the accumulation of amyloid-beta plaques and neurofibrillary tangles in the brain. These pathological hallmarks lead to a cascade of neurochemical imbalances, including disruptions in the cholinergic and glutamatergic systems, both crucial for memory and cognitive function. Current pharmacological interventions for AD focus on modulating these neurotransmitter systems to manage cognitive symptoms and potentially slow disease progression.

Cholinesterase Inhibitors: Boosting Acetylcholine for Enhanced Memory

Cholinesterase inhibitors represent the cornerstone of pharmacological management for mild to moderate AD. These medications work by inhibiting the enzyme acetylcholinesterase (AChE), which is responsible for breaking down acetylcholine (ACh) in the brain. By inhibiting AChE, cholinesterase inhibitors lead to an increase in the synaptic concentration of ACh, a vital neurotransmitter involved in learning, memory, and cognitive processing.

There are three main FDA-approved cholinesterase inhibitors for AD:

Donepezil (Aricept): This medication has a long-lasting effect, typically administered once daily. Donepezil has been shown to improve cognitive function, including memory, attention, and language skills, in individuals with mild to moderate AD.

Rivastigmine (Exelon): Rivastigmine is available in both capsule and patch formulations, offering flexibility in administration. Similar to donepezil, rivastigmine improves cognitive function and may also offer some benefits for behavioral symptoms associated with AD.

Galantamine (Razadyne): This cholinesterase inhibitor has a unique mechanism of action, also acting as a modulator of allosteric sites on nicotinic acetylcholine receptors. Galantamine improves cognitive function and may have some additional benefits for attention and processing speed in individuals with mild to moderate AD.

Benefits and Considerations for Cholinesterase Inhibitors:

While cholinesterase inhibitors cannot halt the progression of AD, they can provide significant benefits for individuals with the disease. Studies have shown improvement in cognitive function, daily living skills, and overall quality of life. However, it's important to consider some key aspects:

Individualized Treatment: The optimal choice of cholinesterase inhibitor and dosage needs to be individualized based on the patient's response and tolerability.

Gradual Response: The benefits of cholinesterase inhibitors may not be immediately apparent. It typically takes weeks or months to observe a noticeable improvement in cognitive function.

Side Effects: Common side effects of cholinesterase inhibitors include nausea, vomiting, diarrhea, and abdominal cramps. Dosage adjustments or alternative medications may be necessary to manage these side effects.

Memantine (Namenda): Modulating Glutamate for Improved Function

Memantine (Namenda) represents another class of medication used for managing cognitive symptoms in moderate to severe AD. Unlike cholinesterase inhibitors, memantine does not directly affect acetylcholine levels. Instead, it works by regulating the glutamatergic system. Glutamate is the brain's most abundant excitatory neurotransmitter, and excessive glutamate activity can be neurotoxic in AD. Memantine acts as an N-methyl-D-aspartate (NMDA) receptor antagonist, modulating glutamate signaling and preventing excitotoxicity.

Benefits and Considerations for Memantine:

Memantine offers some distinct advantages in the management of AD:

Complementary Action: Memantine can be used alone or in combination with cholinesterase inhibitors, potentially offering broader benefits for cognitive function.

Improved Function: Studies suggest that memantine may improve cognitive function, daily living activities, and behavioral symptoms in individuals with moderate to severe AD.

Tolerability: Memantine is generally well-tolerated, with fewer side effects compared to cholinesterase inhibitors.

Limitations of Current Medications:

It is important to acknowledge that both cholinesterase inhibitors and memantine are symptomatic treatments. They do not address the underlying pathology of AD and cannot cure the disease. Furthermore, the effectiveness of these medications can vary significantly between individuals, and some patients may experience minimal cognitive improvement.

The Future of Pharmacological Management:

Research efforts are ongoing to develop new and more targeted medications for AD. These include anti-amyloid and anti-tau therapies that aim to address the hallmark pathologies of the disease. Additionally, exploring combination therapies that target different neurotransmitter systems or disease mechanisms may offer more comprehensive management strategies in the future.

Non-pharmacological interventions and therapies

Cognitive Stimulation Therapy: Rekindling the Spark in Alzheimer's Disease

Alzheimer's disease (AD) is a progressive neurodegenerative disorder that gradually diminishes cognitive function, impacting memory, thinking, and reasoning skills. While there is currently no cure for AD, several interventions can help manage symptoms and improve quality of life for individuals living with the disease. Cognitive stimulation therapy (CST) emerges as a promising non-pharmacological approach, offering a way to "rekindle the spark" by engaging cognitive abilities and promoting social interaction. This section delves deeper into the principles of CST, exploring its benefits for individuals with AD.

The CST Framework: Engaging the Mind in a Supportive Environment

CST is a structured therapeutic approach delivered in small group settings, typically involving 5-7 individuals with AD. Sessions are usually held twice a week for 45 minutes, lasting for several weeks or months. A trained therapist facilitates the sessions, creating a safe and supportive environment where individuals can participate actively. The core principles of CST include:

Structured Activities: Each session revolves around a specific theme, such as current events, reminiscing about the past, or planning a fictional event. Structured activities centered on the theme are used to stimulate cognitive domains like memory, attention, language, and problem-solving skills. These activities can involve group discussions, memory games, puzzles, creative tasks like storytelling or crafts, or even singing familiar songs.

Individualized Approach: Activities are tailored to the individual's cognitive abilities and interests. The therapist adapts the complexity of tasks and provides prompts or cues as needed, ensuring everyone can participate meaningfully.

Social Interaction: CST fosters social interaction and engagement among participants. This allows individuals with AD to connect with others, share experiences, and feel a sense of belonging. Engaging in group discussions also encourages verbal communication skills and expression.

Reality Orientation: Sessions often incorporate elements of reality orientation, where the therapist provides information about the date, time, and location. This can help individuals with AD maintain a sense of time and place.

Benefits of CST: Beyond Cognitive Enhancement

Growing research evidence supports the positive impact of CST on various aspects of well-being in individuals with mild to moderate AD:

Improved Cognitive Function: Studies have shown that CST can lead to measurable improvements in cognitive function, including memory, attention span, and language skills. Engaging in stimulating activities may help maintain cognitive flexibility and strengthen existing neural pathways.

Enhanced Communication Skills: The emphasis on group discussions and shared activities promotes verbal communication skills. Individuals may experience improvement in expressing themselves clearly, following conversations, and engaging in meaningful dialogue.

Elevated Mood and Well-being: Participating in CST can stimulate the release of neurotransmitters like dopamine and serotonin, which contribute to feelings of well-being and social connection. Furthermore, the supportive group environment and successful task completion can boost self-esteem and mood.

Reduced Behavioral Symptoms: CST can indirectly influence behavioral symptoms associated with AD, such as anxiety or agitation. Engaging in stimulating activities and social interaction can redirect attention away from negative thoughts and provide a sense of purpose.

Improved Quality of Life: The combined benefits of CST on cognition, communication, mood, and behavior can significantly enhance the overall quality of life for individuals with AD. This can also alleviate stress and caregiver burden.

Optimizing the Impact of CST: Tailoring Therapy and Considering Limitations

While CST offers numerous advantages, it's crucial to consider some aspects for optimal implementation:

Tailoring Therapy: The therapist needs to assess individual cognitive strengths and weaknesses to tailor activities and ensure an appropriate level of challenge.

Stage of Disease: CST is typically most effective in mild to moderate stages of AD. As the disease progresses, the complexity of activities may need to be adjusted to maintain engagement.

Adherence and Motivation: Regular participation is essential for maximizing the benefits of CST. Creating a supportive and stimulating group environment can enhance adherence and motivation for individuals attending sessions.

CST in the Bigger Picture: A Complementary Approach

CST should be viewed as a complementary approach to managing AD, not a stand-alone treatment. It can be integrated alongside pharmacological interventions, such as cholinesterase inhibitors, to achieve a more comprehensive management strategy. Furthermore, CST can be combined with other non-pharmacological interventions like physical activity, social engagement, and caregiver education to optimize well-being for individuals with AD.

Social Engagement and Activities: Connecting and Maintaining Purpose in Alzheimer's Disease

Alzheimer's disease (AD) is a neurodegenerative disorder that progressively affects memory, thinking, and reasoning skills. However, the impact of AD extends beyond cognitive decline, often leading to social withdrawal and isolation. This can have a profound effect on emotional well-being and exacerbate the progression of the disease. Fortunately, fostering social engagement and activities plays a crucial role in maintaining cognitive and emotional well-being in individuals with AD. This section explores the multifaceted benefits of social engagement and how it can help individuals with AD connect with others, maintain a sense of purpose, and enhance overall quality of life.

The Power of Connection: Combating Isolation and Fostering Well-being

Social isolation is a common concern for individuals with AD. As memory decline progresses, communication difficulties may arise, leading to withdrawal from social interactions. This can have detrimental effects on mood, self-esteem, and cognitive function. Encouraging social engagement and activities provides opportunities for:

Meaningful Interaction: Participating in social activities allows individuals with AD to connect with others, share experiences, and feel a sense of belonging. This social interaction can stimulate conversation and communication skills, keeping them mentally active and engaged.

Reduced Stress and Anxiety: Social connection provides emotional support and reduces feelings of loneliness and isolation. This can improve mood and well-being, potentially reducing stress and anxiety often associated with AD.

Cognitive Stimulation: Social interaction, even in simple forms like reminiscing about the past or engaging in light conversation, can be cognitively stimulating. It promotes memory retrieval, verbal expression, and active listening skills.

A World of Possibilities: Tailoring Activities to Individual Preferences

The specific social activities and interests will vary depending on the individual's abilities, preferences, and stage of the disease. Here are some examples of how to encourage social engagement in AD:

Family Gatherings: Regular get-togethers with family members can provide a familiar and comfortable environment for social interaction. Reminiscing about shared experiences, looking at old photos, or playing simple games can be enjoyable and stimulating.

Volunteer Work: Volunteering opportunities tailored to physical and cognitive abilities can offer a sense of purpose and accomplishment. Folding laundry at a local shelter or helping with simple tasks in a community garden are activities that can promote social interaction and a sense of contribution.

Religious Services: For individuals who find comfort and meaning in religious faith, attending religious services can provide a sense of community and belonging. Singing hymns, listening to sermons, or participating in prayer can offer spiritual comfort and social interaction.

Music and Art Therapy: Music therapy can be a powerful tool for memory retrieval and emotional expression. Listening to familiar music, singing along, or even participating in simple drumming exercises can be stimulating and enjoyable. Art therapy can also provide a creative outlet for self-expression and social interaction.

Social Groups for Individuals with AD: Support groups specifically designed for individuals with AD can offer a safe space to connect with others facing similar challenges. Sharing experiences, offering support, and participating in group activities can promote a sense of belonging and reduce feelings of isolation.

Beyond Socialization: Maintaining Hobbies and Interests

Engaging in hobbies and interests that bring enjoyment is another vital aspect of social engagement in AD. Participating in activities that were previously pleasurable can offer a sense of accomplishment and purpose, even as the individual's abilities may change. This might involve:

Maintaining Familiar Activities: Encourage continued participation in hobbies like gardening, reading (audiobooks can be a great alternative), listening to music, or watching movies. Even if modifications are necessary, such as gardening with raised beds or watching shorter clips of movies, the act of engaging in a beloved activity can be beneficial.

Adapting Activities: If physical limitations make certain activities challenging, consider adaptations or modifications. For example, if painting becomes difficult, exploring simpler art forms like coloring or using larger brushes may allow continued involvement.

Exploring New Interests: Individuals with AD may be open to trying new activities that are less physically demanding but still stimulating. This could involve learning a new language, joining a book club, or participating in adapted sports programs.

Impact on Patients and Caregivers

A. **Frustration, Anxiety, and Depression: Navigating a Changing World in Alzheimer's Disease**

Alzheimer's disease (AD) is a relentless foe, not only stealing memories but also wreaking havoc on an individual's emotional well-being. As the disease progresses, a complex interplay of factors like loss of independence, cognitive decline, and social isolation can trigger a cascade of negative emotions – frustration, anxiety, and depression. Understanding these challenges and their causes is crucial for providing compassionate care and navigating this ever-changing world with individuals living with AD.

Loss of Independence: A Crumbling Foundation for Self-Esteem

The hallmark feature of AD, the gradual decline in cognitive function, inevitably leads to a significant loss of independence. Individuals who were once self-sufficient in daily activities like dressing, bathing, cooking, or managing finances may now require assistance. This erosion of autonomy can be a major source of frustration and anger. The frustration stems from the inability to perform tasks that were once second nature, while the anger often arises from a sense of helplessness and a loss of control over one's life. Witnessing this decline and requiring assistance can also be emotionally taxing for caregivers, creating a dynamic that necessitates open communication and understanding.

Cognitive Decline and Confusion: A Disorienting Labyrinth

The progressive decline in cognitive function in AD is not just about forgetting names or appointments. It can be a deeply disorienting and frightening experience. Memory lapses and difficulty understanding information can lead to confusion and disorientation. Individuals with AD may struggle to recognize familiar places or faces, adding to the sense of fear and insecurity. This cognitive decline can also manifest as difficulty communicating effectively, further amplifying feelings of isolation and frustration. The unpredictability of the disease, where seemingly straightforward tasks become insurmountable challenges, can further fuel anxiety and apprehension.

Social Isolation and Withdrawal: A Fading Connection

Communication difficulties associated with AD can significantly impede social interaction. Individuals with AD may struggle to find the right words, follow conversations, or express themselves clearly. This can lead to social withdrawal and a sense of isolation. Furthermore, the stigma associated with AD may cause them to withdraw from social settings for fear of embarrassment or judgment. The resulting loneliness and isolation exacerbate feelings of depression and contribute to a decline in overall well-being.

A Vicious Cycle: Emotions Feeding on Each Other

These negative emotions often feed into one another, creating a vicious cycle. Frustration from the loss of independence can lead to anger and outbursts. Anxiety triggered by cognitive decline can manifest as sleep disturbances, further impacting cognitive function and fueling depression. Social withdrawal due to communication difficulties can exacerbate feelings of loneliness and isolation, intensifying depressive symptoms.

Breaking the Cycle: Strategies for Emotional Support

Fortunately, there are strategies that caregivers and family members can employ to help individuals with AD manage these negative emotions and navigate this challenging emotional landscape:

Maintaining Routines and Structure: Providing a predictable daily routine with structured activities can provide a sense of security and control, reducing anxiety.

Validation and Empathy: Acknowledging and validating feelings of frustration, fear, or sadness promotes emotional well-being. Using simple language and empathetic communication can ease anxiety and foster a sense of connection.

Focus on Abilities, Not Limitations: Highlighting remaining abilities and focusing on what the individual can still achieve can boost self-esteem and motivate participation in everyday activities.

Promoting Social Interaction: Encourage social interaction in safe and supportive environments. This may involve connecting with family members, participating in support groups, or engaging in activities tailored to the individual's interests.

Maintaining Physical Health: Regular physical activity and a healthy diet contribute not only to physical well-being but also have a positive impact on mood and emotional regulation.

Seeking Professional Help: When Self-Management Isn't Enough

In some cases, the emotional challenges associated with AD may require professional intervention. Mental health professionals can provide individual or group therapy to manage anxiety, depression, and behavioral changes. Furthermore, medications like antidepressants or anti-anxiety drugs can offer additional support for managing these psychological and emotional symptoms.

By creating a supportive environment, employing effective communication strategies, and seeking professional help when necessary, caregivers and family members can play a vital role in helping individuals with AD navigate the emotional challenges associated with the disease. Providing emotional support and fostering a sense of connection can make a significant difference in their quality of life, even as the disease progresses.

B. The Weight of Care: Burden and Challenges Faced by Alzheimer's Disease Caregivers

Alzheimer's disease (AD) is a progressive neurodegenerative disorder that not only affects the individual diagnosed but also significantly impacts their loved ones, particularly those who take on the role of caregivers. Providing care for someone with AD can be an immensely rewarding yet emotionally draining and physically demanding experience. Caregivers often face a multitude of burdens and challenges, impacting their emotional well-being, physical health, and social life. This section explores the various burdens faced by AD caregivers and highlights potential strategies for navigating these challenges.

The Ever-Expanding Role: Juggling Responsibilities and Sacrifices

As AD progresses, the individual's ability to perform daily activities like self-care, managing finances, or medication adherence diminishes. This necessitates a gradual shift in responsibility, placing the caregiver at the center of the caregiving journey. The initial responsibilities may involve assistance with basic needs like bathing, dressing, and meal preparation. Over time, the caregiver's role may expand to include managing finances, medical appointments, communication with healthcare professionals, and navigating legal and social services. This juggle of responsibilities can be overwhelming, particularly when balanced with the caregiver's own work and family commitments.

Emotional Rollercoaster: Navigating Grief, Loss, and Frustration

Witnessing a loved one decline cognitively and emotionally is a heart-wrenching experience for caregivers. Grief for the person they once knew, coupled with the constant fear of future decline, can take a significant emotional toll. Frustration with behavioral changes, communication difficulties, and challenging situations can exacerbate these emotions. Caregivers may also experience feelings of guilt or inadequacy, questioning their ability to provide optimal care.

The Physical Toll: Sleep Deprivation, Stress, and Health Risks

The demands of caregiving can have a detrimental impact on the caregiver's physical health. Disrupted sleep patterns due to nighttime wandering or behavioral issues are common. The physical exertion of assisting with daily activities can lead to fatigue and muscle strain. Chronic stress associated with caregiving weakens the immune system and increases the risk of developing health problems like high blood pressure, heart disease, and depression.

Social Isolation and Strained Relationships:

The time and energy dedicated to caregiving often leave little room for maintaining social connections. Caregivers may withdraw from social activities and hobbies, leading to feelings of isolation and loneliness. Furthermore, the demands of caregiving can put a strain on relationships with family and friends who may not fully understand the challenges faced.

Financial Strain: The Hidden Burden of Care

The financial burden of caring for someone with AD can be significant. Out-of-pocket expenses for medications, in-home care services, or specialized equipment can add up quickly. Caregivers may need to reduce work hours or leave the workforce entirely, further impacting their financial security.

Strategies for Supporting Caregivers: Sharing the Load and Fostering Resilience

While the challenges faced by caregivers are substantial, there are resources and strategies available to support them and promote well-being:

Seeking Support Groups: Connecting with other caregivers facing similar challenges can provide a sense of community, emotional support, and valuable advice. Sharing experiences and learning coping mechanisms can be immensely helpful.

Respite Care: Utilizing respite care services allows caregivers to take a temporary break and recharge. This can be in the form of in-home care services or respite stays in specialized facilities.

Self-Care Practices: Prioritizing self-care practices like getting enough sleep, maintaining a healthy diet, and engaging in regular physical activity is essential for caregivers' physical and mental well-being.

Open Communication: Talking openly with family members and friends about the challenges faced can help them provide emotional support and practical assistance.

Financial Resources: Exploring government assistance programs, long-term care insurance options, or financial aid from non-profit organizations can help mitigate the financial burden.

The Role of Healthcare Professionals:

Healthcare professionals play a crucial role in supporting caregivers by:

Providing education and guidance on managing AD symptoms, behavioral changes, and daily care tasks.

Identifying and addressing caregiver stress, anxiety, and depression.

Connecting caregivers with support groups, respite care services, and community resources.

Advocating for policies that support caregivers financially and offer greater access to resources.

C. Coping Strategies for Patients and Caregivers with Alzheimer's Disease

Alzheimer's disease (AD) is a progressive neurodegenerative disorder that casts a long shadow, impacting not only the individual diagnosed but also their loved ones, particularly those who take on the role of caregivers. While there is currently no cure for AD, a multifaceted approach incorporating coping strategies can significantly improve the quality of life for both patients and caregivers. This section explores effective strategies for managing the emotional, cognitive, and social challenges associated with AD.

Empowering Patients: Maintaining a Sense of Purpose and Engagement

For individuals with AD, the diagnosis can be overwhelming and trigger feelings of fear, anxiety, and frustration. However, implementing coping strategies can help them maintain a sense of control, purpose, and well-being:

Maintaining Routines and Structure: Providing a predictable daily routine with structured activities offers a sense of security and reduces anxiety. This can include familiar mealtimes, bedtime rituals, and participation in preferred activities.

Focus on Abilities, Not Limitations: Highlighting remaining abilities and focusing on what the individual can still achieve can boost self-esteem and motivate participation in daily activities. Occupational therapists can assist in identifying and adapting activities to promote continued independence.

Cognitive Stimulation Activities: Engaging in cognitive stimulation activities like puzzles, memory games, or reminiscing can help maintain cognitive function and provide a sense of accomplishment. Music therapy and art therapy can also be beneficial in promoting emotional expression and cognitive stimulation.

Physical Activity and Exercise: Regular physical activity, tailored to individual abilities, can improve mood, sleep quality, and cognitive function. Maintaining a healthy diet also contributes to overall well-being.

Validation and Empathy: Caregivers should acknowledge and validate feelings of frustration, fear, or sadness. Using simple language and empathetic communication can ease anxiety and foster a sense of connection.

Supporting Caregivers: Building Resilience and Managing Stress

The demands of caring for someone with AD can be emotionally exhausting and physically draining. Caregivers can adopt these strategies to navigate the challenges and build resilience:

Seeking Support Groups: Connecting with other caregivers facing similar challenges can provide a sense of community, emotional support, and valuable advice. Sharing experiences and learning coping mechanisms can be immensely helpful.

Respite Care: Utilizing respite care services allows caregivers to take a temporary break and recharge. This can be in the form of in-home care services or respite stays in specialized facilities.

Self-Care Practices: Prioritizing self-care practices like getting enough sleep, maintaining a healthy diet, and engaging in regular physical activity is essential for caregivers' physical and mental well-being. Practicing relaxation techniques like meditation or deep breathing can also help manage stress.

Open Communication: Talking openly with family members and friends about the challenges faced can help them provide emotional support and practical assistance. Delegating tasks and asking for help can alleviate some of the burden.

Financial Planning: Exploring government assistance programs, long-term care insurance options, or financial aid from non-profit organizations can help mitigate the financial burden of caregiving.

Shared Strategies: Fostering Communication and Connection

Effective communication is vital for both patients and caregivers in navigating the challenges of AD. Here are some strategies to bridge the communication gap:

Simple Language and Repetition: Using simple, clear language and repeating information as needed can enhance understanding and reduce frustration.

Focus on Nonverbal Communication: Facial expressions, body language, and maintaining eye contact can convey emotions and messages beyond words.

Validation and Empathy: Actively listening to patients' concerns and acknowledging their feelings fosters a sense of connection and reduces anxiety.

Maintaining a Calm and Positive Attitude: A calm and positive demeanor from caregivers can create a more relaxed and supportive environment.

Focusing on Shared Activities: Participating in enjoyable activities together, even if adapted to accommodate the patient's abilities, can strengthen the bond and create positive memories.

Seeking Professional Support: Optimizing Care and Well-being

Both patients and caregivers can benefit from seeking professional support:

Individual and Group Therapy: Therapists can provide tools for managing anxiety, depression, and behavioral changes in patients with AD. Caregivers can also benefit from individual or group therapy to address stress, grief, and emotional challenges.

Educational Programs: Educational programs for caregivers can provide valuable information on managing AD symptoms, behavioral changes, and daily care tasks.

Social Services: Social services professionals can help connect patients and caregivers with community resources, support services, and financial assistance programs.

By adopting coping strategies, fostering communication, and seeking professional support, individuals with AD and their caregivers can navigate the challenges of the disease with greater resilience and maintain a sense of well-being.

D. Current Research Trends and Breakthroughs in Alzheimer's Disease

Alzheimer's disease (AD), a neurodegenerative disorder characterized by progressive cognitive decline, poses a significant challenge for healthcare systems worldwide. Despite the absence of a definitive cure, the field of AD research is experiencing a surge in activity, fueled by advancements in technology and a deeper understanding of the disease's underlying mechanisms. This section explores current research trends and recent breakthroughs that offer hope for the future of AD prevention, diagnosis, and treatment.

Targeting the Hallmarks of AD: A Multifaceted Approach

Researchers are increasingly focusing on the underlying pathological hallmarks of AD, including the buildup of amyloid plaques and tau tangles in the brain. These abnormal protein aggregates are believed to disrupt neural communication and contribute to neuronal death. Current research trends explore therapeutic strategies aimed at:

Amyloid-Targeting Therapies: Monoclonal antibodies designed to clear amyloid beta plaques have been a major focus. While some clinical trials have shown promising results in reducing plaque burden, others have yielded mixed outcomes. Researchers are refining targeting strategies and exploring combination therapies with other approaches.

Tau-Targeting Therapies: Research into tau protein aggregation is gaining momentum. Developing drugs that inhibit tau aggregation or promote its clearance holds promise for slowing disease progression.

Neuroinflammation: Chronic inflammation in the brain is increasingly recognized as a key player in AD. Anti-inflammatory drugs are being investigated for their potential to modulate the inflammatory response and protect neurons.

Beyond Plaques and Tangles: Exploring Other Avenues

While amyloid and tau remain central to AD research, investigators are also exploring other potential contributing factors:

Vascular Health: The link between vascular health and cognitive decline is well-established. Research is ongoing to understand how vascular dysfunction contributes to AD and explore interventions that promote healthy blood flow to the brain.

Gut Microbiome: The gut microbiome, the complex ecosystem of microbes in the gut, is gaining attention for its potential role in brain health. Studies are investigating how the gut microbiome might influence AD development and whether manipulating it could offer therapeutic benefits.

Lifestyle Interventions: The focus on modifiable risk factors like diet, exercise, and cognitive stimulation continues. Research is exploring how lifestyle modifications can help prevent or delay AD onset and improve cognitive function.

Revolutionizing Diagnosis: Early Detection for Better Management

Early diagnosis of AD is crucial for effective management and optimizing patient care. Current research delves into:

Biomarkers: Identifying reliable biomarkers in blood, cerebrospinal fluid, or brain imaging scans could enable earlier and more accurate diagnosis of AD.

Artificial Intelligence (AI) and Machine Learning: AI algorithms are being developed to analyze brain scans and identify subtle changes suggestive of early AD. This holds promise for earlier detection and personalized treatment plans.

Emerging Technologies: Advancing Treatment Options

Technological advancements are opening doors for novel therapeutic approaches:

Gene Therapy: Gene therapy techniques aim to modify genes implicated in AD to prevent the production of harmful proteins or enhance neuron protection. While still in early stages, gene therapy holds significant potential for future treatment.

Optogenetics: This technique uses light to stimulate specific neurons. While in pre-clinical stages, optogenetics offers a potential approach to modulate brain activity and improve cognitive function.

Neurostimulation Techniques: Transcranial magnetic stimulation (TMS) and deep brain stimulation (DBS) are being explored for their potential to improve cognitive function and alleviate some of the behavioral symptoms of AD.

Breakthroughs on the Horizon: A Glimpse into the Future

Recent findings offer a sense of optimism for the future of AD research:

Combination Therapies: The recognition of AD's multifaceted nature suggests that combination therapies targeting multiple pathological pathways may be more effective than single-drug approaches.

Precision Medicine: Tailoring treatment plans to an individual's specific genetic and biological profile offers the potential for personalized medicine in AD, maximizing treatment efficacy and minimizing side effects.

Preventative Strategies: As researchers gain a deeper understanding of AD risk factors, the development of preventative strategies to delay or even prevent the disease altogether becomes a possibility.

The Road Ahead: Challenges and Opportunities

Despite the exciting advancements, significant challenges remain. Replicating promising results from pre-clinical studies in human trials, ensuring the affordability of new treatments, and addressing the ethical considerations of emerging technologies are just some of the hurdles that need to be overcome.

E. Advocacy and Awareness Efforts in Alzheimer's Disease

Alzheimer's disease (AD), a relentless neurodegenerative disorder, casts a long shadow, impacting not only individuals diagnosed but also their families and communities. With an aging population and the rising prevalence of AD, the need for public awareness and advocacy efforts has never been greater. This section explores various initiatives aimed at raising awareness, promoting public understanding, and influencing policy changes to support those affected by AD.

Shining a Light on the Disease: Building Public Awareness

Public awareness campaigns play a crucial role in educating the public about AD, its symptoms, and its impact on individuals and families. These campaigns strive to:

Increase Knowledge and Understanding: Raising awareness about the early warning signs of AD can empower individuals to seek early diagnosis and treatment.

Reduce Stigma: Combating social stigma associated with dementia, including AD, is essential. Educational campaigns can promote empathy and understanding, fostering a more supportive environment for individuals living with the disease.

Mobilize Resources: Increased public awareness can garner support for research initiatives, advocacy efforts, and funding for social services and support programs for AD patients and caregivers.

Several strategies are employed to raise public awareness of AD:

Public Service Announcements (PSAs): Utilizing television, radio, and online platforms to broadcast PSAs can effectively reach a broad audience and raise awareness about AD symptoms and available resources.

Media Campaigns: Engaging with media outlets and journalists to share stories of individuals and families living with AD can personalize the impact of the disease and build public empathy.

Community Events: Organizing walks, marathons, or fundraising events can raise awareness, promote community engagement, and generate resources for research and care initiatives.

Social Media Campaigns: Leveraging the power of social media platforms can spread awareness about AD, foster connections among individuals affected, and provide a platform for sharing information and resources.

Advocating for Change: Empowering Voices

Advocacy efforts play a vital role in influencing policy decisions and securing resources for research, care, and support services for those affected by AD:

Lobbying Efforts: Advocacy groups work to influence government policies at local, state, and federal levels. This includes lobbying for increased research funding, improved access to healthcare services for individuals with AD, and support programs for caregivers.

Grassroots Movements: Empowering individuals affected by AD to become advocates for the cause can create a powerful grassroots movement. Sharing personal stories and experiences can influence policymakers and garner public support.

Collaborations: Building partnerships with healthcare professionals, research institutions, and other organizations working on AD can amplify advocacy efforts and lead to more effective outcomes.

Challenges and Opportunities: Navigating the Advocacy Landscape

The path of AD advocacy is not without its challenges:

Competing Priorities: Securing funding for AD research and care initiatives can be difficult in a competitive healthcare landscape with numerous pressing needs.

Public Misconceptions: Public misconceptions about AD, its causes, and treatment options can hinder advocacy efforts.

Diversity and Inclusion: Ensuring advocacy efforts address the needs of diverse communities disproportionately affected by AD is crucial.

Despite these challenges, opportunities exist to advance the cause of AD advocacy:

Harnessing Technology: Utilizing online platforms and social media can empower individuals to become advocates, share their stories, and engage in online advocacy campaigns.

Data and Research: Compelling data highlighting the societal and economic burden of AD can influence policy decisions and resource allocation.

Cross-sectoral Collaboration: Building partnerships with government agencies, private institutions, and philanthropic organizations can broaden the impact of advocacy efforts.

www.ingramcontent.com/pod-product-compliance
Lightning Source LLC
Chambersburg PA
CBHW070306230526
45470CB00002B/743

Financial Freedom: A Roadmap to Building Wealth and Passive Income

Copyright 2024 Michael McGuire

All rights reserved. Published in the United States.

No part of this book may be reproduced or transmitted in any form or by any means, electronic or mechanical, including photocopying, recording, or by an information storage and retrieval system — except by a reviewer who may quote brief passages in a review to be printed in a magazine or newspaper — without permission in writing from the publisher.

The information in this book is for educational purposes only. The author does not guarantee results from the practices detailed in this book. The author is not a broker, CPA, certified financial planner, or attorney. This book is not a substitute for professional advice. It is based on the personal experience and research of the author. Please seek your own consultants.

Table of Contents

Contents

- **Financial Freedom: A Roadmap to Building Wealth and Passive Income** 1
  - Table of Contents 2
  - Introduction 3
  - Chapter 1: Understanding Financial Freedom 7
  - Chapter 2: Building a Strong Financial Foundation 11
  - Chapter 3: Budgeting and Saving 16
  - Chapter 4: Debt Management 23
  - Chapter 5: Investing Basics 27
  - Chapter 6: Advanced Investment Strategies 30
  - Chapter 7: Building Passive Income Streams 34
  - Chapter 8: Real Estate Investments 37
  - Chapter 9: Stock Market Investments 41
  - Chapter 10: Alternative Investments 44
  - Chapter 11: Tax Strategies for Investors 47
  - Chapter 12: Retirement Planning 50
  - Chapter 13: Protecting Your Wealth 53
  - Chapter 14: Case Studies of Financial Success 57
  - Chapter 15: Tools and Resources for Financial Planning 60
  - Conclusion 63